FLUORIDE AND FLUOROSIS

FLUORIDE AND FLUOROSIS

Ashish Sharma BDS PGDPHM
Lecturer
Department of Public Health Dentistry
AMC Dental College
Ahmedabad, Gujarat, India

Foreword

Parthasarathi Ganguly

JAYPEE

JAYPEE BROTHERS MEDICAL PUBLISHERS (P) LTD

New Delhi • London • Philadelphia • Panama

Jaypee Brothers Medical Publishers (P) Ltd

Headquarters

Jaypee Brothers Medical Publishers (P) Ltd
4838/24, Ansari Road, Daryaganj
New Delhi 110 002, India
Phone: +91-11-43574357
Fax: +91-11-43574314
Email: jaypee@jaypeebrothers.com

Overseas Offices

J.P. Medical Ltd
83, Victoria Street, London
SW1H 0HW (UK)
Phone: +44-2031708910
Fax: +02-03-0086180
Email: info@jpmedpub.com

Jaypee-Highlights Medical Publishers Inc
City of Knowledge, Bld. 237, Clayton
Panama City, Panama
Phone: +507-301-0496
Fax: +507-301-0499
Email: cservice@jphmedical.com

Jaypee Medical Inc
The Bourse
111 South Independence Mall East
Suite 835, Philadelphia, PA 19106, USA
Phone: + 267-519-9789
Email: joe.rusko@jaypeebrothers.com

Jaypee Brothers Medical Publishers (P) Ltd
17/1-B Babar Road, Block-B, Shaymali
Mohammadpur, Dhaka-1207
Bangladesh
Mobile: +08801912003485
Email: jaypeedhaka@gmail.com

Jaypee Brothers Medical Publishers (P) Ltd
Shorakhute, Kathmandu, Nepal
Phone: +00977-9841528578
Email: jaypee.nepal@gmail.com

Website: www.jaypeebrothers.com
Website: www.jaypeedigital.com

Inquiries for bulk sales may be solicited at: jaypee@jaypeebrothers.com

Fluoride and Fluorosis

First Edition: **2014**

ISBN: 978-93-5090-855-6

Printed at : S. Narayan & Sons

Foreword

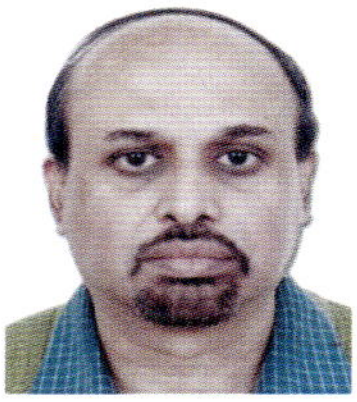

It gives me immense pleasure to know that Dr Ashish Sharma has taken up the endeavor to present his research work in the form of a book. Fluorosis is a significant public health problem affecting millions of people. It has a great adverse effect on the economy of the family, community and country as a whole as it produces partial to total disability. Moreover, with the development of technology, more groundwater is used for drinking and agriculture, and it aggravates the problem of fluorosis. Unfortunately, the attention, knowledge and capacity of the policy makers, program managers, and clinicians are found to be grossly inadequate to deal with such a huge problem.

Dr Ashish had done his research quite elaborately to find out how successful the fluorosis mitigation efforts in the community are. He has put on significant efforts with extensive field work for his research. This book *Fluoride and Fluorosis: A Research Review* is not a textbook but based on his research project findings. Hence, it may have some shortcomings but still a comprehensive effort to elucidate the problem in fluorosis and will be a good reading for the program managers, social workers, primary care physicians and any other person who wish to get a glance of this important but neglected public health problem.

Parthasarathi Ganguly
MBBS MD (Preventive and Social Medicine)
Professor
Indian Institute of Public Health-Gandhinagar (IIPHG)
Gandhinagar, Gujarat, India

Message

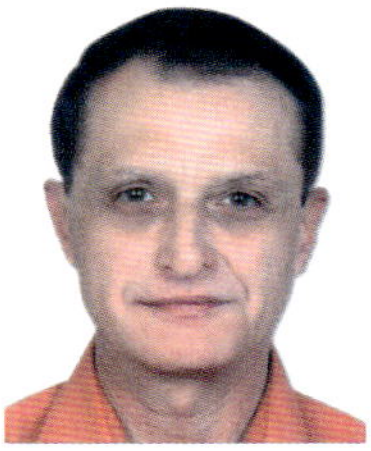

This book provides an insight into the detrimental effects of presence of fluoride in water. The preventive and therapeutic measures have been recommended, which would be essential to educate and inform the affected mass; so as to uplift their overall health and lead a normal life.

Dinyar B Doctor
BDS MDS (Orthodontia)
Former Dean and Head
Department of Orthodontia
AMC Dental College
Ahmedabad, Gujarat, India

Message

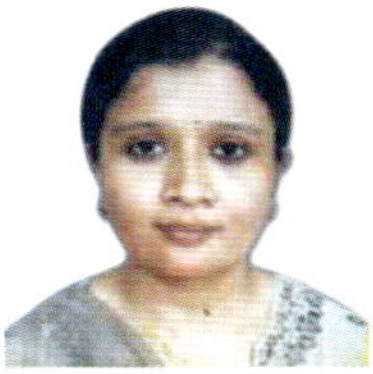

As an academician and an active clinician, I can tell without any doubt that a very important subject is completely neglected by most of the authors of the dentistry and that is the subject of my friend, i.e. *Fluoride and Fluorosis: A Research Review*.

Although fluorosis is such an endemic problem that not much literature exists about it. The genesis of this book is to cater to the lacunae existing in the undergraduate textbooks, which were meant for the postgraduate students. Keeping this as the mission objective, the author has presented a wonderful research and review in a simple and reader-friendly manner. I would appreciate his sincereness and hard working efforts about this neglected subject.

I would definitely recommend it as a must-read book for all dental students and practising dentists.

Anjali Kothari
BDS MDS (Conservative Dentistry and Endodontics)
Head
Department of Conservative,
Endodontics and Esthetic Dentistry
AMC Dental College
Ahmedabad, Gujarat, India

Preface

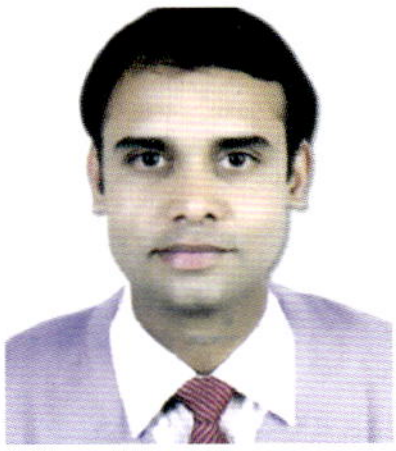

This book is a research review and compilation of authentic facts regarding dental and skeletal fluorosis. It also throws light on what is fluorosis actually, its causative factors and how to detect it clinically and radiologically based on certain parameters. The purpose of this research study was to assess the prevalence of fluorosis and comparing it with previous studies to know the effects of mitigation measures taken to curb fluorosis.

This book throws an insight into the actual picture of fluorosis and ways to detect the fluorosis afflicted people based on proven indices and obvious detectable clinical and radiological parameters. This book will be useful to those who want to further carry out research on fluorosis and the ways to detect the fluorosis afflicted people. This book is an initiative to probe and research into the gravity of the problem of fluorosis and provide critical inputs to them who want to carry out researches to detect fluorosis and furthermore to devise innovative methods to curb it. This book is useful for the undergraduate medical students, public health experts, public health managers, health economists, NGOs, postgraduate (PG) medical students pursuing PG courses in Public Health, and national and international agencies working to eradicate fluorosis. This book also throws a glimpse on the socioeconomic aspect of people with relation to fluorosis.

This book can be an ideal notebook for the medical/dental students who want to understand dental and skeletal fluorosis in clear and simple manner with its explicit contents and noteworthy pictures, tables and diagrams. Simultaneously, this book will be very much handy to those who want to know the methods and concepts to conduct further research on fluorosis.

It is different from other books in terms of relevant and actual description of concept of fluorosis with actual diagrams, colored pictures, tables, figures, charts, graphs and actual data. It is unique in its appearance as diverging from theoretical concept of fluorosis to the research methodological concept of fluorosis enabling to cover the interest of the vast masses of people ranging from students to researchers and professionals up to national and international agencies.

Hence, I am very much grateful to the almighty who gave me strength and courage to publish this book based on actual fieldwork to understand the concept of fluorosis.

Ashish Sharma

Acknowledgments

I take this opportunity with much pleasure to thank all the people, who have helped me through the course of my journey towards producing this review of mine research work. I sincerely thank Dr Parthasarathi Ganguly, Professor, Indian Institute of Public Health-Gandhinagar (IIPHG), for his guidance, help and motivation.

Apart from the subject of my research, I had learnt a lot from him, which I am sure, will be useful in my future career. I would like to express my sincere gratitude to Dr Rajnarayan Indu and Dr Sunderrajan Krishnan of Indian Natural Resource Economics and Management (INREM) Foundation (Carewater), for great help with the research design and methodology. I am also grateful to Dr Deepak Saxena, Assistant Professor, IIPHG, Ahmedabad, who encouraged me to do study on fluorosis.

Special thanks go to Dr AK Susheela, Executive Director of the Fluorosis Research and Rural Development Foundation in India, Professor of Anatomy (Histocytochemistry) and Chief of the Fluoride and Fluorosis Research Laboratories, All India Institute of Medical Sciences, New Delhi, for giving me the tips of doing research study on fluorosis.

I wish to thank my parents, Suresh Chandra Sharma and Sumitra Sharma, whose love, teachings and support have brought me this far. Finally, this thesis would not have been possible without the confidence, endurance and support of my wife Priyanka Sharma, who has always been a source of inspiration and encouragement. I wish to thank my brother Dr Vivek Sharma and my sister Preeti Sharma, and my brother-in-law Dheerendra Upadhyay, for their affection, understanding and patience.

Contents

1. Introduction to Fluorosis **1**

2. Aims and Objectives **41**

3. Literature Review **42**

4. Methodology **46**

5. Inferences **51**

Annexures *75*

Bibliography *93*

Glossary *95*

Index *97*

1

INTRODUCTION TO FLUOROSIS

FLUORINE

Geochemistry of Fluorine

The name fluorine originated from the Latin word 'fluere' (meaning 'to flow'). Fluorine is the 13th most ubiquitous pollutant, abundant on earth. In its elemental form, it is a pale yellow, highly toxic and corrosive gas (Glasser, 1979). French scientists Henri Moissan discovered it in 1886. He has been awarded Nobel Prize in chemistry for this discovery in 1906 (Glasser, 1979). It combines with all elements except oxygen and noble gases to form fluorides. Fluorides are ubiquitous in nature and are present in rocks, soil, water, plants, foods and even air.

Several natural and anthropogenic sources contribute to the geochemical cycling of fluorine. The most important industrial processes that release fluorine compounds are—aluminium smelting, coal burning, phosphate fertilizer and cement production, and brick and ceramic firing. Fluorine is the lightest member of the halogen group and is one of the most reactive of all chemical elements. It is not, therefore, found as fluorine in the environment. It is the most electronegative of all the elements (Hem, 1989) which means that it has a strong tendency to acquire a negative charge, and in solution forms fluoride ions.

Geochemists have established that the fluorine content of the earth's crust is 950 parts per million (ppm), while chlorine content is seven times less than that. Despite that, sea water contains 1.3 mg/L fluoride as against 19,500 mg/L chloride. This indicates that the natural environment of the earth has a favorable mechanism to immobilize toxic fluoride for the safe existence of life.

In the humid, temperate tracts of the world, groundwater is distinctly acidic particularly due to acid rains caused by industrial pollution and contains little fluoride even when local rocks and soils contain high fluorine. People living in such tracts are prone to caries, necessitating fluoridation of drinking water supplies.

In the arid/semiarid tracts of the world including India, groundwater is distinctly alkaline to contain high fluoride even when local rocks and soils contain less fluorine.

People living in such tracts are prone to fluorosis unless provided with low-fluoride drinking water.

If groundwater contains more than 1.0 mg/L of fluoride and is used for a long time for drinking and cooking purpose then it may cause fluorosis in living beings.

Forms of Fluorine

Fluorine can be isolated in two different forms including the molecular, diatomic gas, F_2, and the ionic form, F^-. It is very difficult to isolate fluorine in its atomic form due to its high reactivity and electronegativity.

Reactivity

Fluorine is the most reactive of the halogens. Fluorine is the most electronegative element currently known. This means the elemental form, F, will actively seek another electron to satisfy the octet rule (8 electrons in the outer s and p shells). This extra electron could come from anything. Because of this, fluorine is the strongest known oxidizer. It is only found naturally on earth as ^{19}F, its only stable isotope. Aqueous HF [hydrofluoric acid], is weakly acidic. This acid will dissociate in water, but only to small extent. In its dissociated form, F^-, it is a fairly strong base. Anhydrous HF (hydrogen fluoride) is a strong acid and its strength can be greatly increased through the addition of a lewis acid such as antimony pentafluoride.

Synthesis

Fluorine is not produced in a monatomic, uncharged form. It is generally always manufactured from the mineral fluorite, which is the major source of fluorine on earth. Though it is not produced as an elemental form, fluorine can be produced in its ionic and diatomic gas forms. This is done by a method developed by Henri Moissan in 1886. The method begins by reacting potassium fluoride and hydrogen fluoride, KF and HF respectively, to form potassium hydrogen bifluoride, KHF_2. This compound is produced in an aqueous solution and is further electrolyzed to form gaseous hydrogen, gaseous fluorine, and ionic fluorine in an aqueous solution, H_2, F_2 and F^- respectively.

Reactions

Molecular fluorine will act as an oxidant in most reactions. In electrochemistry, strong oxidizers have a high standard reduction potential. This value refers to the tendency of the compound or element in question to be reduced, or gain electrons. Fluorine has the highest standard reduction potential, +2.87V, making it the strongest oxidizer. Fluorine is known to react violently with hydrogen and alkali metals. It will react with alkali earth metals less violently and may form an insoluble salt. It is also know to form covalent bonds with transition metals, noble gases, and organic compounds. Due to its high reactivity, gaseous fluorine must be kept under dry conditions. If it comes in contact with moisture, it will decompose to form HF gas.

Available Forms

Fluorine can be very dangerous in its gaseous form. However, it is still available for purchase from chemical suppliers around the world. It can also be obtained by the purchase of fluorine containing compounds. It would have to be produced by one method or another of chemical conversion and isolation from these compounds.

FLUORIDE

Introduction

Fluoride is the negatively charged ionic form of the element fluorine that has a high affinity for calcium. In the human body, it is mainly associated with bones and teeth. Fluoride plays a very important role in the prevention of dental caries. Although the primary mechanism of action of fluoride in preventing dental caries is topical, systemic mechanisms are also important.

Fluoride acts in the following 3 ways to prevent dental caries (listed in order of importance):

1. It enhances remineralization of the tooth enamel. This is the most important effect of fluoride in caries prevention.
2. It inhibits demineralization of the tooth enamel. A mineral structure of the tooth that includes fluoride (fluorapatite) is more resistant to demineralization than one without fluoride.
   Hydroxyapatite: A complex phosphate of calcium $Ca_5(PO_4)_3OH$ that occurs as a mineral and is the chief structural element of vertebrate bone.
3 It makes cariogenic bacteria (e.g. streptococcus mutans) less able to produce acid from carbohydrates.

Magnitude of Problem

Distribution

Fluoride in water is mostly of geological origin. Waters with high levels of fluoride content are mostly found at the foot of high mountains and in areas where the sea has made geological deposits. Known fluoride belts on land include—one that stretches from Syria through Jordan, Egypt, Libya, Algeria, Sudan and Kenya, and another that stretches from Turkey through Iraq, Iran, Afghanistan, India, northern Thailand and China. There are similar belts in the Americas and Japan. In these areas fluorosis has been reported.

Fluoride in Water

Since some fluoride compounds in the earth's upper crust are soluble in water, fluoride is found in both surface waters and groundwater. In surface freshwater, however, fluoride concentrations are usually low—0.01 ppm to 0.3 ppm.

In groundwater, the natural concentration of fluoride depends on the geological, chemical and physical characteristics of the aquifer, the porosity and acidity of the soil and rocks, the temperature, the action of other chemical elements, and the depth of wells. Because of the large number of variables, the fluoride concentrations in groundwater can range from well under 1 ppm to more than 35 ppm. In Kenya and South Africa, the levels can exceed 25 ppm. In India, concentrations up to 38.5 ppm have been reported.

Scope of the Problem

The prevalence of dental and skeletal fluorosis is not entirely clear. It is believed that fluorosis affects millions of people around the world, but as regards dental fluorosis the very mild or mild forms are the most frequent.

International Status

The following countries have been identified for the problem of fluorosis: Pakistan, Bangladesh, Argentina, United States of America, Morocco, Middle East countries, Japan, South African Countries, New Zealand, and Thailand, etc.

In India

High groundwater fluoride concentrations associated with igneous and metamorphic rocks such as granites and gneisses have been reported from India, Pakistan, West Africa, Thailand, China, Sri Lanka, and Southern Africa.

In Gujarat

The groundwater of 4341 or 52.6% villages of the total 8252 villages in Gujarat is contaminated with more than 1.5 mg/L of fluoride. But WHO's recommendation for permissible fluoride is 1.0 mg/L. The people of all these villages are under the risk of fluorosis. However, all of them may not be afflicted by fluorosis because it largely depends on the metabolism and the degree of immunity of a person (Shah and Indu).

The geological survey of India has brought out considerable data which reveal that fluorite, topaz, apatite, rock phosphate, phosphatic nodules and phosphorites are widespread in India and contain high percentage of fluorides.

Fluoride is a highly reactive poison, which is not essential in drinking water by any scientific measure. In India, fluorosis was first detected in Nellore district of Andhra Pradesh during early nineteen thirties by farmers. They found it among their cattle. Later they found the same symptoms of ache and pains in joints, etc among themselves and among the people of neighborhood villages. The first medical report on Fluorosis was published during 1937 in the Indian Journal of Medical Research. Since then a lot

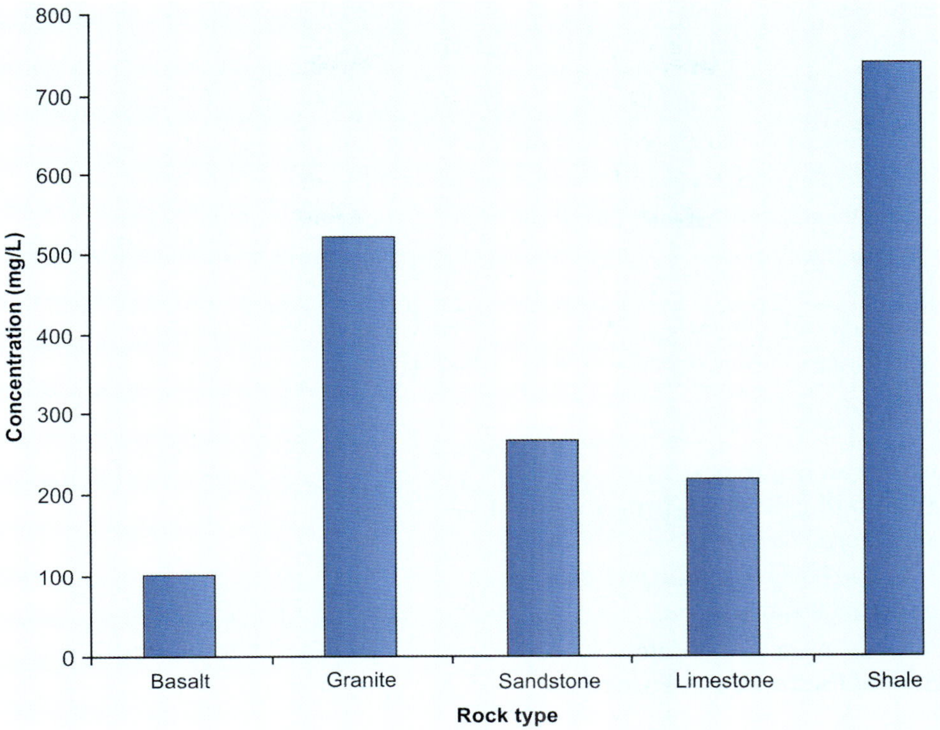

Figure 1.1: Average concentration of fluorine in main rock types
[*Source*: Athavale, R.N. and Das, R.K. (1999). Down to Earth, 8(6): 24-25].

of research work had been published primarily from Andhra and later from many other places of India.

The problem has reached alarming proportions affecting at least 17 states of India. Out of those 5 are hyper endemic, where 50–100% districts are affected viz. Andhra Pradesh, Tamil Nadu, Uttar Pradesh, Gujarat, Rajasthan. Major sources of fluoride for human exposures are water, food, air, medicament and cosmetics. It is roughly estimated that 60% of the total intake of fluoride is through drinking water. In India, it has been observed that tea, fluoridated tooth paste and high fluoride water make a major contribution for human ingestion.

FLUOROSIS

Definition

Fluorosis is a water-borne non-communicable disease. Fluorosis is a disease caused due to excessive ingestion of fluoride in human or animal body. Fluorosis is a crippling and painful disease caused by intake of fluoride. Fluorides are the compounds of fluorine. Fluorine is the 13th most abundant element available in the earth crust. As the surface water passes through the fluoride rich rocks it carries fluoride with it, hence most of the fluoride is found in ground water than surface water.

What is fluorosis and how it can harm you?

- If the presence of fluoride is more than one milligram in one litre water, it is considered harmful
- Consumption of excess fluoride causes three types of fluorosis—dental, skeletal and non-skeletal
- Dental fluorosis can be evident from chalky white teeth and yellow-to-brown pigmentation on teeth
- Skeletal fluorosis leads to anterior bowing of lower limb bones and stiffness to back and neck muscles
- A person with non-skeletal fluorosis has neurological and muscular ailments like weakness, nervousness, tingling sensation to fingers and stiffness.

Source: himalnews.wordpress.com

Fluorosis can occur as:
- Water-borne fluorosis (hydrofluorosis)
- Food-borne fluorosis
- Drug and cosmetic induced fluorosis
- Industrial fluorosis.

Historical Facts about Fluorosis

- In 1866, fluoride was discovered by French scientist Henri Moissan
- In early part of 20th century residents of certain areas of USA developed brown stains on teeth
- In 1925, the term fluorosis was coined and used by Cristian and Guatier
- In 1930, relationship between mottled enamel and fluoride in water was established
- In 1930, Feil mentioned fluorosis in human as an occupational disease
- In 1932, skeletal fluorosis was reported in humans as an occupational disease
- In 1937, skeletal fluorosis was 1st reported in India
- Feil first mentioned fluorosis in humans as an occupational disease in 1930. This was substantiated when the occurrence of skeletal fluorosis in cryolite miners in Denmark was reported (Moller and Gudjonsson 1932). In India, fluorosis was first reported in the then Madras Presidency in 1937.

The Disease and How It Affects People

Ingestion of excess fluoride, most commonly in drinking-water, can cause fluorosis which affects the teeth and bones. Moderate amounts lead to dental effects, but long-term ingestion of large amounts can lead to potentially severe skeletal problems. Paradoxically, low levels of fluoride intake help to prevent dental caries. The control of drinking-water quality is therefore critical in preventing fluorosis.

The Condition and Its Effect on People

Fluorosis is caused by excessive intake of fluoride. The dental effects of fluorosis develop much earlier than the skeletal effects in people exposed to large amounts of fluoride. Clinical dental fluorosis is characterized by staining and pitting of the teeth. In more severe cases all the enamel may be damaged. However, fluoride may not be the only cause of dental enamel defects. Enamel opacities similar to dental fluorosis are associated with other conditions, such as malnutrition with deficiency of vitamins D and A or a low protein-energy diet. Ingestion of fluoride after six years of age will not cause dental fluorosis.

Chronic high-level exposure to fluoride can lead to skeletal fluorosis. In skeletal fluorosis, fluoride accumulates in the bone progressively over many years. The early symptoms of skeletal fluorosis, include stiffness and pain in the joints. In severe cases, the bone structure may change and ligaments may calcify, with resulting impairment of muscles and pain.

Acute high-level exposure to fluoride causes immediate effects of abdominal pain, excessive saliva, nausea and vomiting. Seizures and muscle spasms may also occur.

The Cause

Acute high-level exposure to fluoride is rare and usually due to accidental contamination of drinking-water or due to fires or explosions. Moderate-level chronic exposure (above 1.5 mg/L of water—the WHO guideline value for fluoride in water) is more common. People affected by fluorosis are often exposed to multiple sources of fluoride, such as in food, water, air (due to gaseous industrial waste), and excessive use of toothpaste. However, drinking water is typically the most significant source. A person's diet, general state of health as well as the body's ability to dispose of fluoride all affects how the exposure to fluoride manifests itself. Fluoride ingestion occurs through fluoridated beverages, fluoride-rich foods such as tea, ocean fish, gelatin, skin of chicken, fluoridated salt, food contaminated with fluoride-containing insect or post-harvest fumigants (e.g. sulfuryl fluoride) and pesticides (e.g. cryolite, sodium aluminium fluoride, Na_3AlF_6, which may be used on grapes) etc., fluoridated toothpastes, fluoride from any other environmental source, including cigarette smoke and industrial pollution, e.g. fluoride in dust and fumes from industries such as those manufacturing steel, aluminum, enamel, pottery, glass, bricks, phosphate fertilizer, and others involved with power, welding, water fluoridation plants, refrigeration, rust removal, oil refining, plastics, pharmaceuticals, tooth-paste, chemicals, and automobiles.

Fluoride is ingested from other sources apart from fluoridated water such as pesticides, post-harvest fumigants, air, food, salt, medications, toothpaste, dental restorations, health supplements, medications containing fluoride and fluoride mouth rinses, black rock salt (fluorite, CaF_2) and foods containing black rock salt (Kala Namak) for flavor, e.g. Dhalmoth, other salty snacks, chat masala, etc., red rock salt and foods made using red rock salt and tobacco or supari (Aracanut) when they are chewed by themselves. Regardless of the fluoride ingested by all sources, severity of fluorosis increases with an increase in the malnutrition of people.

GEOGRAPHICAL DISTRIBUTION OF FLUOROSIS IN INDIA

(http://www.downtoearth.org.in/html/20030415_map.htm)

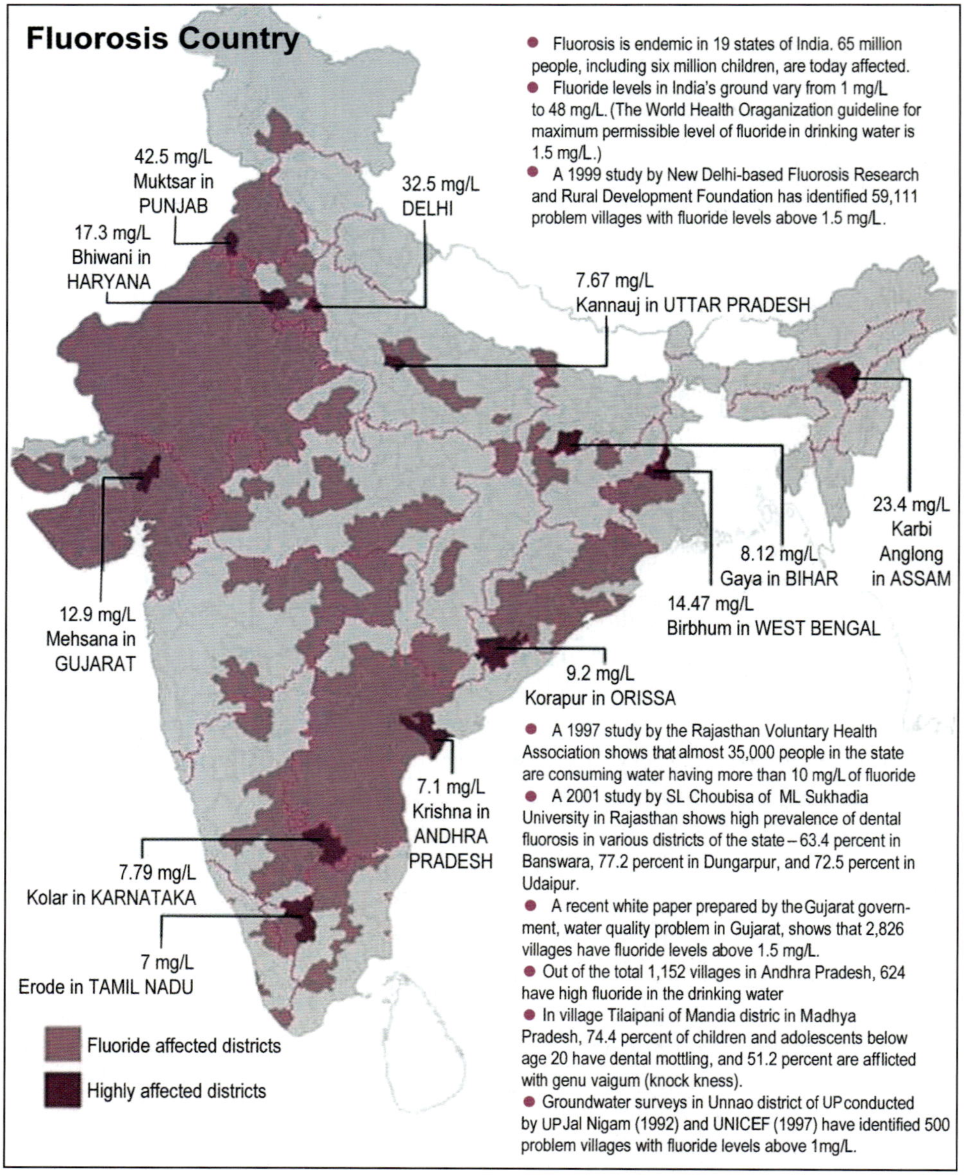

Figure 1.2: Geographical distribution of fluorosis in India

Nevertheless, in the most affected states listed above, half or more of the districts have some villages with ground water supplies having high fluoride concentrations. In these states, 10 to 25 per cent of the rural population has been estimated to be at risk, and perhaps a total of 60–70 million people in India as a whole may be considered to be so (UNICEF, 1999).

Worldwide domestic use of water is about 10% (FAO; 2002b; Crops and Drops); in India, the domestic use is 4.5% (IRMA/UNICEF, 2002) and 'groundwater accounts for nearly 50% of the urban domestic and 80% of the rural domestic water need in India' (Dinesh Kumar et al, 2004).

Long back it was believed that fluorosis is a problem of elderly age group but it have been found that children in the age group of 0 to 12 years are most prone to fluorosis as their body tissues are in formative/growth stage during this period. The problem is so severe that if expectant mothers ingest high fluoride water, it can create many problems with developing fetus. It not only affects the body of a person but also renders them socially and culturally crippled.

The Factors, Which Govern the Development of Fluorosis, are the following

1. High levels of fluoride in drinking water supplies and in the foodstuffs grown in these endemic areas.
2. Tropical weather and hard manual labor by affecting the intake of water.
3. Poor nutrition and diets deficient in their content of calcium, magnesium and vitamin C aggravate fluoride toxicity. High intake of calcium reduces the amount of absorbed into the bones.
4. Magnesium has a peculiar relationship with fluoride and its optimum intake helps in elimination of fluoride from the body. Vitamin C is beneficial in some way in reducing fluoride toxicity. Diets deficient in calories and calcium intake increase the incidence of fluorosis (WHO-2002).
5. Renal disease aggravates fluorosis by increased deposition of fluoride in the bones. A diseased kidney cannot handle fluoride excretion from the body and hence its increased deposition in the bones.
6. Presence of abnormal amounts of certain trace elements in the drinking water supplies such as strontium, uranium, etc. Strontium levels in drinking water supplies in some endemic areas are high and strontium is a bone-seeking element like fluoride and both these aggravate the bony changes.

Diagnosis

Other conditions may look like fluorosis. Developmental defects and problems with the skull or bones of the face can disrupt the enamel or dentin of the teeth. In addition, high fevers or trauma (such as a fall that injures a tooth) in infants or young children may discolor teeth. Young children can get cavities in their primary teeth, so any tooth discoloration should be checked at the dental office.

Differential Diagnoses

The differential diagnosis for this condition may include Turner's hypoplasia (although this is usually more localized), some mild forms of amelogenesis imperfecta, and other environmental enamel defects of diffuse and demarcated opacities. All three types of presentations in fluorosis need to be differentiated from simulating illnesses.

Difficulty in Diagnosing

Fluorosis is a crippling disorder due to entry of fluoride in the body. A proper thorough and in-depth pathological, radiological and physiological diagnosis is necessary before declaring a case or 'stamped' the case, as 'fluorosis' one. It also needs to test the water being used by the patient and to know how long the patient is using the same water. The incubation period of fluorosis is very long. Many symptoms of Fluorosis are somewhat alike with other diseases such as *'Va'*, arthritis, osteoporosis, etc. At the village level, as told by the Medical Officers, it is very difficult to diagnose a patient properly, which requires analysis of X-ray, blood and urine by a good experienced doctor. Hence 'stamped' (the coin word used by the Government Medical Officers, Gujarat) cases of Fluorosis are not available. However, it does not mean that there is no incidence of Fluorosis particularly, when it is known that water is contaminated with fluoride and being used for a long time in the location. Hence cases of fluorosis are mixed with MSD and recorded as general MSD [musculo-skeletal disease] in hospitals and NGO's Health Centers as government did not want to recognize the incidences of fluorosis (Shah and Indu).

Dental Fluorosis

Like any other organs in the body; teeth are also affected by various factors leading to diseases. The differential diagnosis of flluorosis should be done for two aspects:

1. Related to the pitting and chipping in fluorosis
2. Related to discoloration of teeth.

Common Dental Diseases Relating to the Pitting and Chipping in Fluorosis are:

1. Dental caries or decay/cavity formation
2. Periodontal disease or pyorrhea
3. Dental fluorosis.

Caries appear as black spots or cavity in the tooth when decay reaches dentin. Person complains of sensitiveness and acute pain when decay reaches pulp. Pyorrhea is caused by action of bacteria present in the mouth on food, resulting in the form of brownish hard deposit on the surface of teeth near gum. Periodontal disease is the inflammation of gingival gum and periodontal ligament leads to deposition of inorganic salts known as tartar, it irritates gum resulting in bleeding of gums and bad breath. Tartar cannot be removed by brushing. Periodontal disease is more common amongst persons suffering from diabetes mellitus, nutritional deficiency, especially protein and Vitamin C deficiency.

Fluorosis affects permanent teeth though decay of temporary teeth is also reported.

Diseases Related to Discoloration of Teeth

There may be two types of staining of teeth:

a. Internal staining
b. External staining.

Fluorosis causes internal staining of teeth, whereas other causes like brinjal eating, banana biting, palm leaf biting, coconut leaf chewing cause external staining of teeth and may be mistaken for dental fluorosis.

Expected Duration

The spots and stains left by fluorosis are permanent. They may be darken over time.

Permissible Limit of Fluoride

To a certain extent (as per WHO; 0.6 ppm) fluoride ingestion is useful for bone and teeth development, but excessive ingestion causes fluorosis.

WHO and BIS 10500: 1991standards permit only 1.5 mg/L as a safe limit for human consumption. (http://www.krassindia.org/downloads/ebook1.pdf on fluoride and Fluorosis).

The 1984 WHO guidelines suggested that in areas with a warm climate, the optimal fluoride concentration in drinking water should remain below 1 mg/L (1ppm or part per million), while in cooler climates it could go up to 1.2 mg/L. The differentiation derives from the fact that we perspire more in hot weather and consequently drink more water. The guideline value (permissible upper limit) for fluoride in drinking water was set at 1.5 mg/L, considered a threshold where the benefit of resistance to tooth decay did not yet shade into a significant risk of dental fluorosis.

(The WHO guideline value for fluoride in water is not universal: India, for example, lowered its permissible upper limit from 1.5 ppm to 1.0 ppm in 1998.)

CHEMOBIOKINETICS AND METABOLISM OF FLUORIDE

Ingested fluoride is rapidly absorbed through gastrointestinal tract and lungs. Approximately 75–90 per cent of ingested fluoride is absorbed. In an acidic stomach, fluoride is converted into hydrogen fluoride (HF) and up to about 40 per cent of the ingested fluoride is absorbed from the stomach as HF. High stomach pH decreases gastric absorption by decreasing the concentration uptake of HF. Fluoride not absorbed in the stomach is absorbed in the intestine and is unaffected by pH at this site (Whitford, 1997; IPCS, 2002). Relative to the amount of fluoride ingested, high concentrations of cations that form insoluble complexes with fluoride (e.g. calcium, magnesium and aluminium) can markedly decrease gastrointestinal fluoride absorption (Whitford, 1997; IPCS, 2002).

The peaks are reached after 30 minutes in blood. The rapid excretion takes place through renal system over a period of 4 to 6 hours. In children less than 3 years of age only about 50% of total absorbed amount is excreted, but in adults and children over

3 years—about 90% is excreted. Approximately 90% of the fluoride retained in the body is deposited in the skeleton and teeth. The biological half-life of bound fluoride is several years. Fluoride also passes through the placenta and also appears in low concentrations in saliva, sweat, and milk.

Much of the fluoride ingested by human beings is excreted by the kidney, guts and skin and, in the case of women, lost also through menstruation, offspring and lactation.

The toxic effects of fluorine retained by the body are minimal owing to more than 95% of it getting immobilized by substituting for hydroxyl ions in apatite present in dental and skeletal structures (hard tissues) to become fluor-apatite. Although initial entry of fluorine into the hard tissues is beneficial for the health of teeth and bones, entry of more fluorine results in dental and skeletal fluorosis. Once fluorine levels in the hard tissues reach physiologic saturation, which ranges from 0.02 to 0.83%, further ingestion of fluoride leads to flooding of fluoride in the soft tissues leading to skin, urinary, gastric, muscular and neurological problems, besides death due to some intercurrent infection.

Fluoride added to water supplies is a byproduct of the manufacture of superphosphate and aluminum. It is also a byproduct of manufacture of steel, lead, copper, and nickel. Fluoride is quite toxic and was once widely used in insecticides and rodenticides. Goodman and Gilman write, "The pharmacological actions of fluoride, with the possible exception of its effect on bone and teeth, can be classified as toxic.

Of great concern is what has been termed the "Genetic Toxicity of Fluoride." Fluoride causes chromosome aberrations in plants. Chromosome aberrations have also been observed in animal and human cell cultures. One study concludes that "the weight of the evidence leads to the conclusion that F^- (fluoride) exposure results in chromosome aberrations.

Mechanism of action

The best way to view the mechanism of action by which fluorine breaks down bones and causes skeletal fluorosis is in a step-wise fashion.

1. Fluorine enters the body by two paths: Ingestion or respiration. Both paths lead to corrosion of exposed tissue in high concentrations. Since the most likely form of Fluorine to enter the body is hydrogen fluoride gas, this is what starts the process. Exposed tissues will be utilized by HF in neutralization reactions.
2. This will leave F^- free to pass further into the body.
3. It reacts with the concentrated HCl in the stomach to form the weak acid, HF.
4. This compound is then absorbed by the gastrointestinal tract and passes into the liver via the portal vein. Since F is the strongest oxidizer known currently, it is immune to phase 1 metabolic reactions, which are generally oxidation reactions, in the liver. These reactions are the body's first line of defense to biotransform harmful compounds into something more hydrophilic and more easily excreted.
5. The HF is now free to pass into the blood stream and be distributed to all tissues including bones.
6. Bones are largely composed of Ca compounds, particularly carbonated hydroxyapatite ($Ca_{10}(PO_4)_6(OH)_2$); the reaction of Ca and HF forms an insoluble salt, CaF_2.
7. This salt must be cleared by the body and as a result washes away some of the calcium that would be part of the bone matrix.
8. This process results in increased density, but decreased strength in bones.

The mechanism of how fluoride does its damage is now fairly well understood. Fluoride can form a strong bond with protein structures within living systems. Fluoride has a very strong affinity for hydrogen. Hydrogen is the major molecule which links DNA together. "Thus some of the serious charges that are being laid at its door—genetic damage, birth defects, cancer and allergy response—may arise from fluoride interference after all."

Fluoride interferes with the formation of normal collagen, the protein cement which holds body structures together. Total collagen is increased, as much as 50% in one study, but the collagen is imperfect. Structures heavily dependent upon collagen include tooth enamel and dentin, bone, cartilage, and muscle and skin. Teeth could be more heavily mineralized, while being imperfect. This is what we appear to see with water fluoridation.

Fluoride also appears to disturb mineralization and may contribute to mineralization of soft tissues.

Distribution

- 96–99% of fluoride retained in body combines with mineralized bones
- When the ingestion is >5 mg, 50% is retained by skeleton and the rest is excreted through urine
- Normal plasma fluoride levels are 0.14–0.19 PPM in non-endemic areas
- Fluoride levels in soft tissues are < 1PPM, in brain 0.4–0.68 PPM, in CSF it is 0.1 PPM
- Fluoride uptakes is faster in young bones
- Fluoride content in skeletal bones varies, it is highest in bones of pelvis and vertebrae.

Excretion of Fluorides

1. *Feces*

Fluoride present in feces results from two sources—the ingested fluoride that is not absorbed and the absorbed fluoride that is excreted into the gastrointestinal tract. About 10–25% of daily intake of fluoride is excreted in the feces.

2. *Urinary*

The elimination of absorbed fluoride occurs almost exclusively via the kidneys. Urinary fluoride in normal individuals fluctuates widely between 0 and 1.2 PPM with an average of about 0.4 PPM when fluoride content of drinking water is 0.3PPM. Urinary levels of fluoride are higher in individuals exposed to higher intake of fluoride. The renal clearance of fluoride is directly related to urinary pH, and under some conditions, to urinary flow rate. In alkaline urine the fluoride is present in ionic form and hence its renal clearance is rapid. In the acidic urine on the other hand, fluoride is present in nonionic form (HF) and hence it is rapidly reabsorbed in renal tubules. The excretion of fluoride is much less if person concerned is suffering from chronic kidney disease resulting in renal failure, which inevitably leads to high concentrations of fluoride in serum as well as bone.

3. *Sweat*

Some fluoride is also lost from the body through sweat and so appreciable amounts may be lost in situations marked by excessive sweating. Sweat fluoride concentrations are similar to plasma.

4. *Other Routes*

The amount of fluoride in breast milk is low and same is true of saliva.

Table 1.1: Effect of Fluoride concentration on teeth

Fluoride concentration (mg/L)	*Effect*
Nil	Limited growth and fertility
< 0.5	Dental caries
0.5–1.5	Promotes dental health, prevents tooth decay
1.5–4.0	Dental fluorosis (mottling and pitting of teeth)
4.0–10.0	Dental fluorosis, skeletal fluorosis (pain in neck bones and back)
> 10.00	Crippling fluorosis

Source: International Drinking Water Standards (1971), WHO, Geneva

Physiology

Dental fluorosis occurs because of the excessive intake of fluoride, either through fluoride in the water supply, naturally occurring or added to it; or through other sources. The damage in tooth development occurs between the ages of 3 months to 8 years, from the overexposure to fluoride. Teeth are generally composed of hydroxyapatite and carbonated hydroxyapatite; when fluoride is present, some fluorapatite is generated. Excessive fluoride can cause white spots, and in severe cases, brown stains or pitting

Fluoride and bone cells—notable quotes:

1. "The changes which occur in chronic fluorosis, such as mottling of teeth and skeletal effects, are probably secondary to cellular disfunction, caused by toxic levels of fluoride in the vicinity of the cells. This interference of cell function may be related to inhibitory effects of fluoride on specific enzyme systems." *Source*: Cimasoni G. (1970). Fluoride and enzymes. In: TL Vischer, ed. (1970). Fluoride in Medicine. Hans Huber, Bern. pp. 14–26.
2. "At a certain level of fluorine intake the metabolism of the bone tissue is altered and the balance between osteoblastic and osteoclastic activity may be upset."
   Source: Rockert H. (1963). X-ray absorption and X-ray fluorescence micro-analysis of mineralized tissue of rats which have ingested fluoridated water. Acta Pathologica et Microbiologica Scandinavica 59: 32–38.
3. "It was concluded that the observed changes cannot be explained by F induced changes in a single cell. Fluoride appears to affect all cells involved in remodeling by direct or indirect mechanisms." *Source*: Kragstrup J, et al. (1989). Effects of fluoride on cortical bone remodeling in the growing domestic pig. Bone 10:421–424.
4. "Because fluoride injures all of the cells involved in bone formation and degradation, it is not surprising that a poor quality of bone accumulates in patients treated with fluoride." *Source*: Krook L, Minor RR. (1998). Fluoride and alkaline phosphatase. Fluoride 31: 177–182.

or mottling of enamel. Fluorosis cannot occur once the tooth has erupted into the oral cavity. At this point, fluorapatite is beneficial because it is more resistant to dissolution by acids (demineralization). Although, it is usually the permanent teeth which are affected, occasionally the primary teeth may be involved.

Long back it was believed that fluorosis is a problem of elderly age group but it have been found that children in the age group of 0 to 12 years are most prone to fluorosis as their body tissues are in formative/growth stage during this period. The problem is so severe that if expectant mothers ingest high fluoride water, it can create many problems with developing fetus. It not only affects the body of a person but also renders them socially and culturally crippled.

FLUORIDE TOXICITY

In high concentrations, soluble fluoride salts are toxic and skin or eye contact with high concentrations of many fluoride salts is dangerous. Referring to a common salt of fluoride, sodium fluoride (NaF), the lethal dose for most adult humans is estimated at 5 to 10g (which is equivalent to 32 to 64 mg/kg elemental fluoride/kg body weight). A toxic dose that may lead to adverse health effects is estimated at 3 to 5 mg/kg of elemental fluoride. Ingestion of fluoride can produce gastrointestinal discomfort at doses at least 15 to 20 times lower (0.2–0.3 mg/kg) than lethal doses. Although helpful for dental health in low dosage, chronic exposure to fluoride in large amounts interferes with bone formation. In this way, the greatest examples of fluoride poisoning arise from fluoride-rich ground water.

Quantification of Fluoride Toxicity on Human Health

Smith and Hodge have related the concentrations or doses of fluoride to the biological effects indicated in the tabulation below:

Table 1.2: Effect of fluoride toxicity on human health

Fluoride concentration (mg/L)	*Source*	*Effects*
0.002	Air	Destructive effect on plants
1.00	Water	Prevention of dental caries
≥ 2	Water	Affect dental enamel
≥8	Water	Affect bones and muscles
>50	Food and water	Changes in thyroid
>100	Food and water	Defective development
>120	Food and water	Changes in kidney

Acute Toxicity

Mechanism

Like most soluble materials, fluoride compounds are readily absorbed by the stomach, intestines and excreted through the urine. Urine tests have been used to ascertain rates of excretion in order to set upper limits in exposure to fluoride compounds and associated detrimental health effects. Ingested fluoride initially acts locally on the intestinal mucosa, where it forms hydrofluoric acid in the stomach. Thereafter it binds calcium and interferes with various enzymes.

Sources

Historically, most cases of fluoride toxicity have followed accidental ingestion of sodium fluoride based insecticides or rodenticides. Currently, in advanced countries most cases of fluoride exposure are due to the ingestion of dental fluoride products. Although exposure to these product does not often cause toxicity.

Organofluorine Compounds

Organofluorine compounds only rarely release F^- under biological conditions and thus are rarely sources of fluoride poisoning. In order for fluoride poisoning to occur, a compound must release fluoride (F^-) ions. Whereas most organofluorine compounds may not release F^- because of the strength of the carbon-fluorine bond and its tendency to strengthen as more fluorine atoms are added to a carbon, others do, such as methoxyflurane. The fluorine atom is pervasive in drugs, e.g. prozac, and many other substances such as freon, teflon, and blood serum (PFOS, PFOA, and PFNA).

Symptoms

Poisoning comes from ingesting a large amount of fluoride in a short period of time. Ingesting 3-5 mg/kg may cause symptoms to appear, while the estimated lethal dose is 5-10 g (32-64 mg/kg) in adults and 16 mg/kg in children. Severity of symptoms depends upon the amount of fluoride ingested. These include abdominal pain, diarrhea, dysphagia, hypersalivation, mucosal injury, nausea, vomiting. Electrolyte abnormalities including hyperkalemia, hypocalcemia, hypoglycemia, and hypomagnesemia may occur. Neurological symptoms include headache, muscle weakness, hyperactive reflexes, muscular spasms, paresthesia seizures, tetanic contractions, and tremors. In severe cases, multi-organ failure will occur. Death typically results from cardiac arrest, shock, widening of QRS, and various arrhythmias occur.

Fluoride in Toothpaste

Children may experience gastrointestinal distress upon ingesting sufficient amounts of flavored toothpaste. Gastrointestinal symptoms appear to be the most common problem reported.

Treatment of Acute Toxicity

1. Monitor and support vital signs, including cardiac monitoring
2. Gastric lavage, if emesis has not occurred. Charcoal is probably not of benefit
3. Monitor serum electrolyte, calcium, and magnesium levels
4. Treat hypocalcemia, hypomagnesemia and hyperkalemia or hypokalemia
5. Administer milk, oral calcium salts, or aluminum or magnesium based antacids to bind fluoride
6. Consider hemodialysis in patients with significant toxicity
7. Treat arrhythmia, especially in the presence of refractory hyperkalemia
8. Consult a regional poison center for the latest treatment recommendations.

Chronic Toxicity

In India an estimated 60 million people have been poisoned by well water contaminated by excessive fluoride, which is dissolved from the granite rocks. The effects are particularly evident in the bone deformations of children. Similar or larger problems are anticipated in other countries including China, Uzbekistan, and Ethiopia.

Although fluoride may be present in a medication or an anesthetic agent, it may be less toxic by being in a bound rather than a free form. Unless fluorinated organic chemicals are metabolized in the body to release the fluoride they contain, the covalently bound fluoride may be eliminated from the body without having been released as free fluoride ions. A small increase in the serumd fluoride level occurs with the partially metabolized ciprofloxacin, a fluoroquinolone antibiotic, while a larger increase occurs with fluorinated anesthetics such as halothane, which are metabolized to a greater extent. It is possible that small amounts of fluoride released from fluoride-containing medications may be a cause of illness, particularly if the release is in an area, such as the brain, where even minute concentrations may have a very potent effect.

Symptoms of Chronic Fluoride Poisoning

1. Chronic fatigue not relieved by extra sleep or rest
2. Headaches
3. Dryness of the throat and excessive water consumption
4. Frequent need to urinate
5. Urinary tract irritation
6. Aches and stiffness in muscles/bones (sarthritic like pain), in lower back, in neck area, in jaws, in arms, shoulders and legs
7. Muscular weakness
8. Muscles spasms (involuntary twitching)
9. Tingling sensations in fingers (especially) and feet
10. Gastrointestinal disturbances:

    The intestinal lining or mucosa of the duodenal region normally has cells with small protrusions on them (microvilli) and a layer of slimy substance (mucus). The microvilli and mucus are lost with chronic fluoride toxicity giving rise to symptoms such as nausea, loss of appetite, pain in the stomach, gas formation and a bloated feeling, constipation followed by intermittent diarrhea, and headache. These symptoms of non-ulcer dyspepsia are early warning signs of fluoride toxicity.

- Abdominal pains
- Diarrhea
- Constipation
- Blood in stools
- Bloated feeling (gas)
- Tenderness in stomach area
- Feeling of nausea (flu like symptoms)

11. Pinkish red or bluish red spots (like bruises but round or oval) on the skin that fade and clear up in 7–10 days
12. Loss of mental acuity and ability to concentrate
13. Depression
14. Excessive nervousness
15. Dizziness
16. Tendency to lose balance
17. Visual disturbances like Temporary blind spots in field of vision and diminished ability to focus (possible retinal damage)
18. Brittle nails
19. Repeated miscarriages or still births
20. **Male infertility**: Male infertility with abnormalities in sperm morphology, a deficiency in the number of spermatozoa in the semen (oligospermia), the absence of spermatozoa from the semen (azoospermia), and low testosterone levels are very common in those residing in areas of India where chronic fluoride toxicity is common due to fluoride-contaminated water
21. Dental fluorosis with discoloration of the enamel of the front teeth, the central or lateral incisors of the upper and lower jaws.

The only generally accepted adverse effect of fluoride at levels used for water fluoridation is dental fluorosis, which can alter the appearance of children's teeth during tooth development; this is mostly mild and usually only an aesthetic concern.

Consumption of fluoride at levels beyond those used in fluoridated water for a long period of time causes skeletal fluorosis. In some areas, particularly the Asian subcontinent, skeletal fluorosis is endemic. It is known to cause irritable-bowel symptoms and joint pain. Early stages are not clinically obvious, and may be misdiagnosed as (seronegative) rheumatoid arthritis or ankylosing spondylitis.

Other adverse effects may be possible at fluoride intake levels above the recommended dosage, and defluoridation is recommended in these cases.

Excess Fluoride Consumption has been Studied as a Factor in the following

- A weakening of bones, leading to an increase in hip and wrist fracture.
- Adverse effects on the kidney. Within the recommended dose, no effects are expected, but chronic ingestion in excess of 12 mg/day are expected to cause adverse effects, and an intake that high is possible when fluoride levels are around 4 mg/L. Those with impaired kidney function are more susceptible to adverse effects.
- Fluoride's suppressive effect on the thyroid is more severe when iodine is deficient, and fluoride is associated with lower levels of iodine. Thyroid effects in humans were associated with fluoride levels 0.05–0.13 mg/kg/day when iodine intake was adequate and 0.01–0.03 mg/kg/day when iodine intake was inadequate.

CLINICAL MANIFESTATIONS OF FLUOROSIS

Fluoride has beneficial effects on teeth at low concentrations in drinking-water, but excessive exposure to fluoride in drinking-water, or in combination with exposure to fluoride from other sources, can give rise to a number of adverse effects. These range from mild dental fluorosis to crippling skeletal fluorosis as the level and period of exposure increases. Crippling skeletal fluorosis is a significant cause of morbidity in a number of regions of the world.

Toxic Effects on Human Beings

Fluorosis may cause skeletal fluorosis, dental fluorosis, non-skeletal manifestations, or any combination of the above and in final stages it causes premature aging.

Dental Fluorosis

Dental Fluorosis is the most convenient biomarker of exposure to fluoride. Dental fluorosis is a reflection of what's happening in our bones and is the first visible sign of fluoride poisoning.

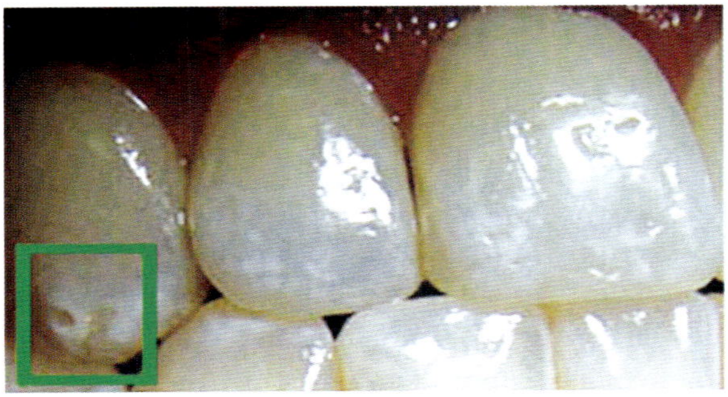

Figure 1.3: Dental fluorosis

Source: http://www.cosmetic-dentistry-center.com/fluorosis-a-250.html

It is defined as a change in the mineralization of the dental hard tissues (enamel, dentin, and cementum) caused by long-term ingestion (eating and drinking) of fluoride during the period of tooth development prior to eruption into the mouth (first 8 years of life for most permanent teeth excluding third molars). Once the tooth erupts, dental fluorosis refers to a range of visually detectable changes in enamel. The severity of dental fluorosis depends on when and for how long the overexposure to fluoride occurs, the individual response, weight, degree of physical activity, nutritional factors and bone growth, suggesting that similar dose of fluoride may lead to different levels of dental fluorosis.

Other factors that may increase the individual susceptibility to dental fluorosis are:

- Altitude
- Malnutrition
- Renal insufficiency.

Dental fluorosis is a developmental disturbance of dental enamel, caused by successive exposures to high concentrations of fluoride during tooth development, leading to enamel with lower mineral content and increased porosity. The severity of dental fluorosis depends on when and for how long the overexposure to fluoride occurs, the individual response, weight, degree of physical activity, nutritional factors and bone growth. The risk period for esthetic changes in permanent teeth is between 20 and 30 months of age.

The recommended level for daily fluoride intake is 0.05–0.07mgF/kg/day, which is considered of great help in preventing dental caries, acting in remineralization. A daily intake above this safe level leads to an increased risk of dental fluorosis.

Dental fluorosis is a known adverse effect of fluoride overuse. Enamel or dental fluorosis is a condition caused by 'excessive' intake of fluoride over an extended period of time.

As described by Cutress and Suckling, the first clinical signs of dental fluorosis are thin white striae across the teeth surfaces. These fine opaque lines seem to follow the perikymata pattern. The cusp tips, incisal edges and marginal ridges may appear completely opaque, a condition that has been defined as "snow-capping." In moderately affected teeth, the white lines appear more pronounced. The lines may merge and produce areas that will appear cloudy and will be scattered over the tooth surface. With increasing severity, the entire surface exhibits opaque, cloudy areas that may be mixed with areas of brownish discoloration. In the most severe cases, pitting of the enamel surface occurs. The most common symptom of dental fluorosis is a chalk-like discoloration of teeth with white spots or lines on tooth enamel. In more severe cases, the affected areas have a yellow or brown discoloration. In extreme forms, fluorosis may result in a pitted tooth surface.

Fluorosis is a cosmetic problem and not a dental disease. Teeth are strong and healthy, but the spots and stains left by fluorosis are permanent and may darken over time. Dental fluorosis can be cosmetically treated by a dentist by microabrasion or tooth bleaching.

Dental or enamel fluorosis occurs only while the teeth are still developing under the gums, before their eruption. Dental fluorosis occurs during the development of the tooth, with permanent teeth being more susceptible than primary teeth. Further, dental fluorosis is less prevalent and less severe in the primary teeth than in the permanent dentition.

The most critical ages of susceptibility are from 0 to 6 years, especially between the ages of 15 and 30 months (15–24 months for boys, 21–30 months for girls). After 7 or 8 years of age, dental fluorosis cannot occur because the permanent teeth are fully developed, although not erupted.

Fluoride causes dental fluorosis by damaging the cells that form the enamel, called ameloblasts. Damage to these cells results in a mineralization disorder of the teeth, whereby the porosity of the sub-surface enamel is increased. Fluorosis occurs when fluoride interacts with mineralizing tissues, causing alterations in the mineralization process. In dental enamel, fluorosis causes subsurface hypomineralizations or porosity, which extend toward the dentinal-enamel junction as severity increases. This subsurface porosity is most likely caused by a delay in the hydrolysis and removal of enamel proteins, particularly amelogenins, as the enamel matures. This delay could be due to the direct effect of fluoride on the ameloblasts or to an interaction of fluoride with the proteins or proteinases in the mineralizing matrix. The specific mechanisms by which fluoride causes the changes leading to enamel fluorosis are not well defined; though the early-maturation stage of enamel formation appears to be particularly sensitive to fluoride exposure. The development of fluorosis is highly dependent on the dose, duration and timing of fluoride exposure. The risk of enamel fluorosis is lowest when exposure takes place only during the secretory stage, but highest when exposure occurs in both secretory and maturation stages. The incidence of dental fluorosis is best correlated with the total cumulative fluoride exposure to the developing dentition. Fluoride supplements can contribute to the total fluoride exposure of children, and if the total fluoride exposure to the developing teeth is excessive, fluorosis will result.

Fluoride consumption can exceed the safe dose when a child drinks a lot of fluoride containing water in combination with other dietary fluoride sources (foods with high fluoride content), or by just swallowing fluoridated toothpaste.

Dental fluorosis is a health condition caused by a child receiving too much fluoride during tooth development. The critical period of exposure is between 1 and 4 years old; children over age 8 are not at risk. Dental fluorosis can develop in children but not in adults. Dental fluorosis in an adult is a result of high fluoride exposure when the adult was a child or adolescent. Teeth with fluorosis also have an increased porosity of the enamel. Even with mild fluorosis, enamel is subject to increased erosion and attrition because the structural integrity of enamel is compromised. As enamel breaks away, small pits are become visible. In the milder forms, the porosity is

Dental fluorosis

- Mainly involves enamel
- Mottling is one of the earliest in most recognizable feature
- Both sexes are equally affected
- Permanent teeth are affected
- Teeth become rough, opaque and chalky white
- Pitting and chipping also occurs
- In endemic areas dental fluorosis has linear relationship to fluoride content of water

mostly limited to the sub-surface enamel, whereas in the more advanced forms, the porosity impacts the surface enamel as well, resulting in extensive pitting, chipping, fracturing and decay of the teeth.

The discoloration induced by fluorosis—particularly in its advanced forms—can cause significant embarrassment and stress to the impacted child, resulting in adverse effects on esteem, emotional health, and career success.

White opacities, faint yellow stain, pitting, chipped off, black discoloration, enamel hypoplasia, delayed eruption, etc. may result due to dental fluorosis. The incidences of mottled teeth were observed even with range of 0.7–1.5 mg F/L in drinking water. The minimal daily fluoride intake in infants that may cause very mild or mild fluorosis in human beings was estimated to be about 0.1 mg per kg body weight. The severity of dental fluorosis depends on the amount of fluoride exposure, the age of the child, individual response, as well as other factors including nutrition. Although water fluoridation can cause fluorosis, most of this is mild and not usually of esthetic concern. Severe cases can be caused by exposure to water that is naturally fluoridated to levels well above the recommended levels, or by exposure to other fluoride sources such as brick tea or pollution from high fluoride coal. Teeth may show dental caries with cavities when drinking water has less than around 1 mg/L. Teeth are generally free of caries and fluorosis when fluoride is around 1 mg/L. Mild dental fluorosis is developed when fluoride is in between 1 and 2.5 mg/L.

Severe dental fluorosis is developed when fluoride is more than 2.5 mg/L.

Epidemiologic Indices

Several indices have been used to describe the clinical appearance of dental fluorosis. The three principal epidemiologic indices used for measuring the clinical manifestations of dental fluorosis which are in use nowadays are—those developed **by Dean (1934, 1942), Thylstrup and Fejerskov (1978), and Horowitz et al. (1984) and a recent index (Fluorosis Risk Index) developed by Pendrys (1990).**

The continued use of Dean's classification system and derived index (CFI) for more than a half century is testimony to its simplicity and utility. The index has been criticized because the unit of analysis is the person, because criteria are unclear for some categories, or that they lack sensitivity, particularly for severe fluorosis, and because of the way in which data are summarized and reported. The Thylstrup and Fejerskov Index is appealing to clinicians and epidemiologists alike in that it corresponds closely to histological changes that occur in dental fluorosis and to enamel fluoride concentrations, thereby having biological validity. The TSIF described by Horowitz, et al. makes a useful contribution because it provides clearer diagnostic criteria and provides for an analysis based on esthetic concerns. The Fluorosis Risk Index appears to be particularly useful for analytical epidemiologic studies, because it is designed to permit a more accurate identification of associations between age-specific exposures to fluoride and the development of dental fluorosis. All three indices in common use today provide useful indices for the study of dental fluorosis. The utility of the Fluorosis Risk Index will be determined as it receives wider use. The selection of one of these indices for use in an epidemiologic study depends in large measure on the purpose of the study. Research needs to continue on the validity of these indices, particularly for mild fluorosis, and on the public's perception of the cosmetic appearance of teeth with different severity levels of fluorosis.

Histology

The histological examination shows hypomineralized, porous sub-surface enamel below a well mineralized surface layer. The most affected teeth (in decreasing order) are premolars, 2nd molars, followed by maxillary incisors, canines and 1st molars. Mandibular incisors are affected least.

Following are the Vital Criterias to Determine Dental Fluorosis:

- Discoloration of the teeth with a pattern
- Discoloration horizontally aligned/never vertical
- Discoloration away from the gums
- Discoloration is bilaterally symmetrical.

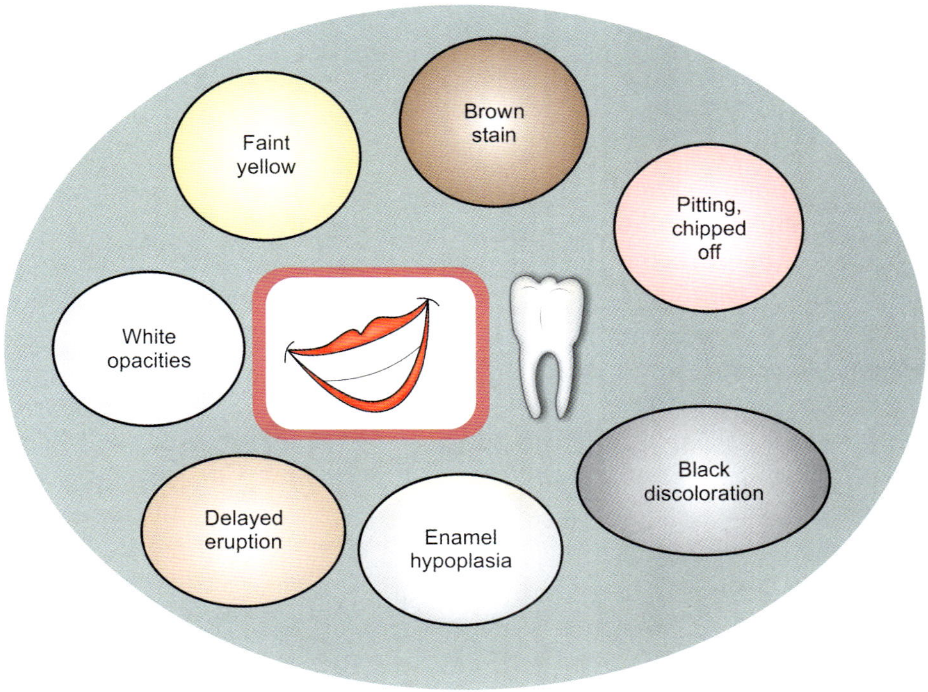

Figure 1.4: Different criterias to determine dental fluorosis

Grades of Fluorosis

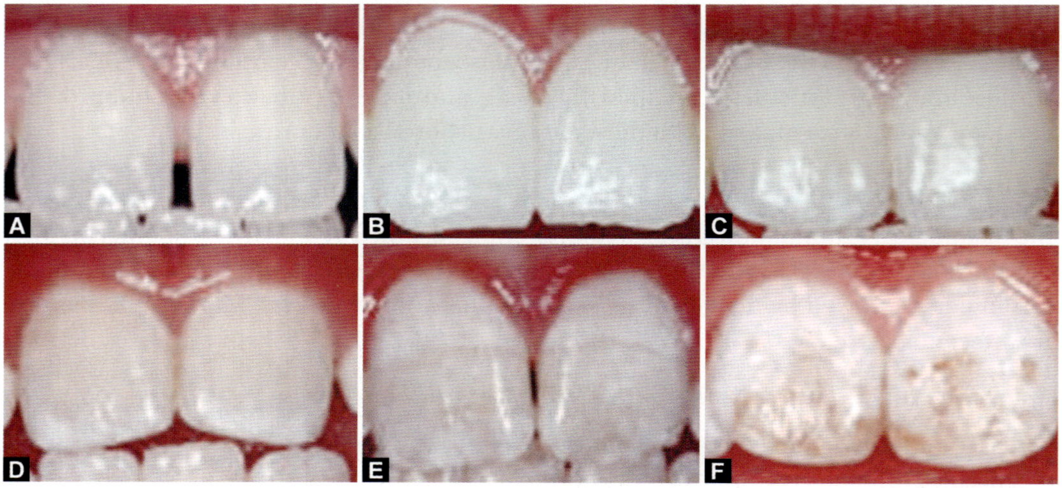

Figures 1.5Ato F: (A) Normal; (B) Questionable; (C) Very mild; (D) Mild; (E) Moderate; (F) Severe
Source: http://www.cdc.gov/fluoridation/safety/dental_fluorosis.htm

Severe Dental Fluorosis

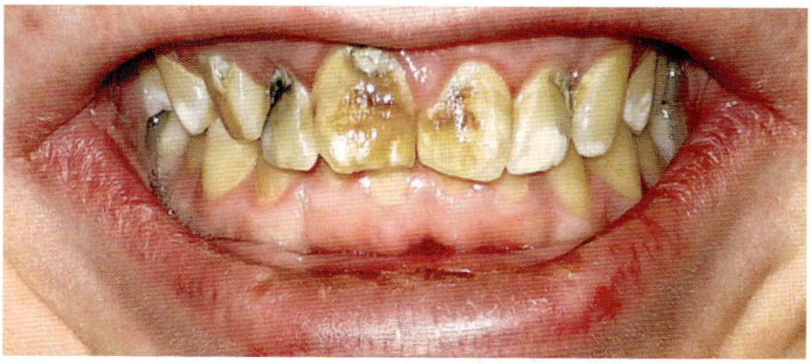

Figure 1.6: Severe dental fluorosis
Source: http://en.wikipedia.org/wiki/Dental_fluorosis

Dental Fluorosis

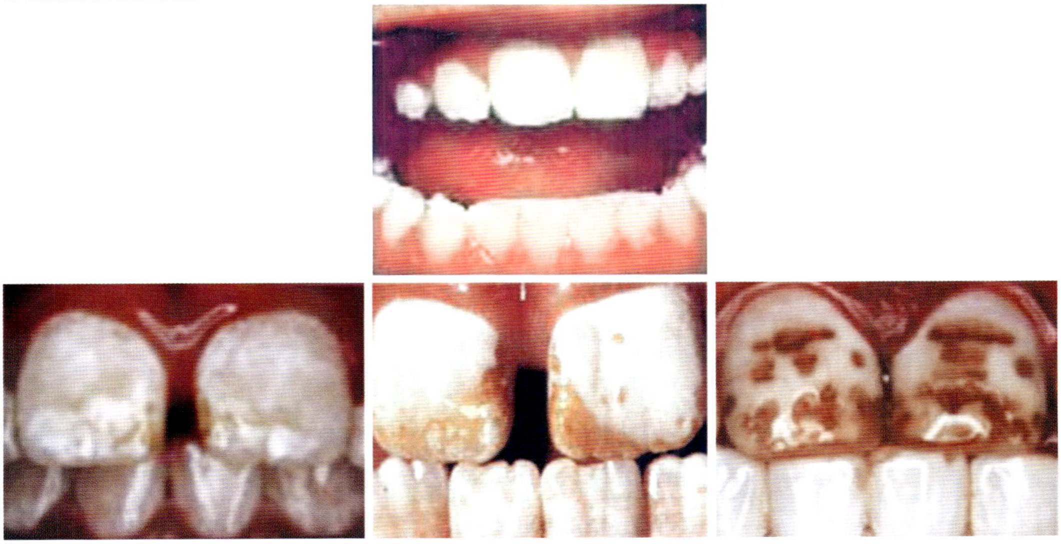

Figure 1.7: Dental fluorosis
Source: The public perception of dental fluorosis
George Glasser and Jane Jones* http://g-tigerclaw.com/mm/percdf.htm

Grades of Dental Fluorosis

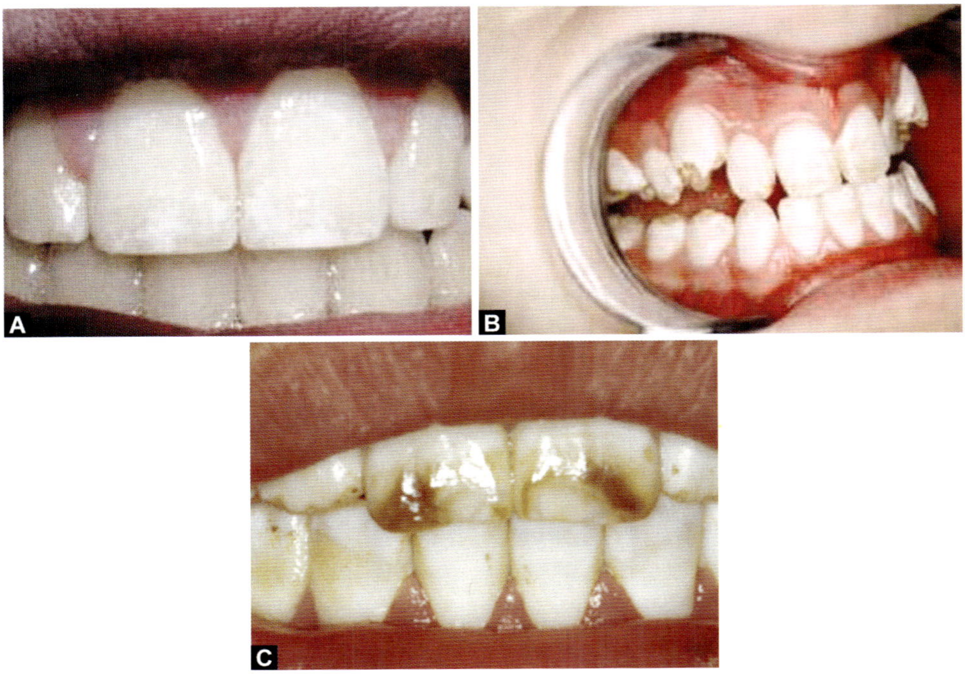

Figures 1.8A to C: (A) Mild dental fluorosis; (B) Severe dental fluorosis; (C) Moderate dental fluorosis
Source: http://www.waterloowatch.com/Index_files/Fluoride%20and%20Dental%20Fluorosis.pdf

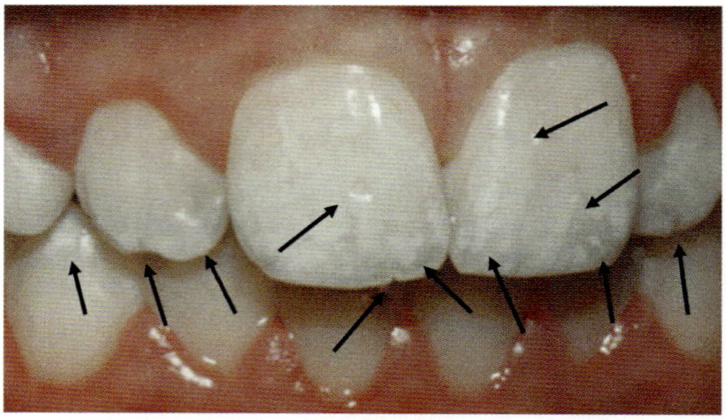

Figure 1.9: Moderate effects of fluoridated water. Arrow point to discolored, cracked or pitted areas
Source: http//clouddragon.files.wordpress.com/2009/12/dental-fluorosis.gif

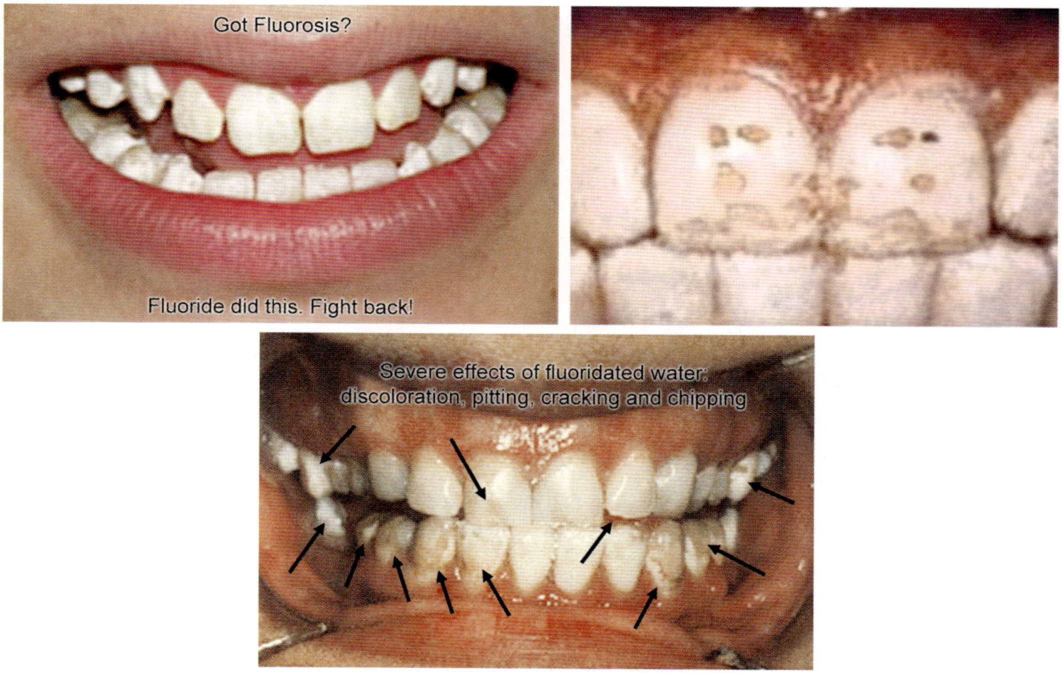

Figure 1.10: Fluorosis arising from exessive fluoride content in water
Source: http://www.google.co.in/search?q=Fluorosis+photographs&hl=en&prmd=ivns&tbm=isch&tbo=u&source =univ&sa=X&ei=_mGyTbDhE4vtrQf189XIDQ&ved=0CBsQsAQ&biw=1259&bih=399

Picture of Dental Fluorosis

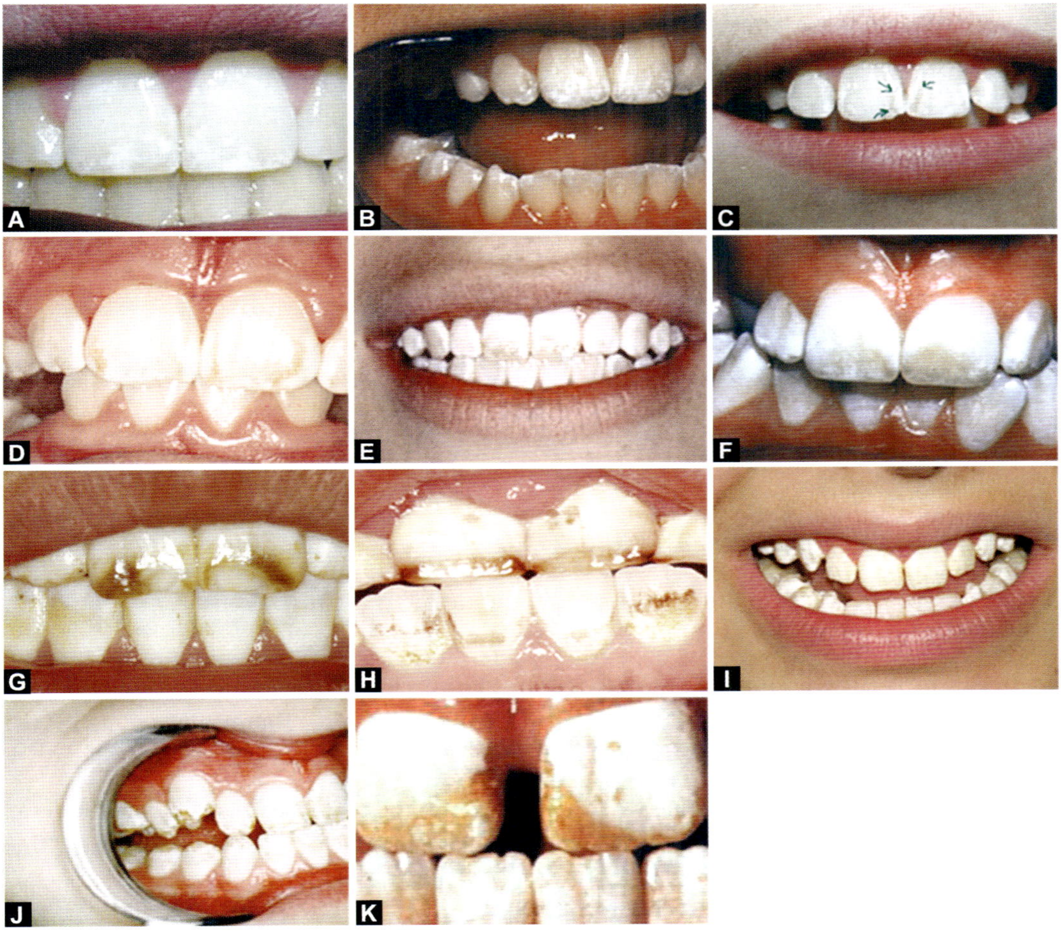

Figures 1.11A to K: (A) Mild fluorosis (*Photo by Hardy Limeback, DDS*); (B) Mild fluorosis (*Photo by Elke Babiuk*); (C) Mild fluorosis (*Photo by Hardy Limeback, DDS*); (D) Mild fluorosis (*Photo by David Kennedy, DDS*); (E) Mild fluorosis (*Photo by Jeffrey Hamilton, DDS*); (F) Mild/moderate fluorosis (*Photo by Elke Babiuk*); (G) Moderate/severe fluorosis (*Photo by David Kennedy, DDS*); (H) Moderate/severe fluorosis (*Photo by David Kennedy, DDS*); (I) Severe fluorosis (*Photo by Hardy Limeback, DDS*); (J) Severe fluorosis (*Photo by Hardy Limeback, DDS*); (K) Severe fluorosis (*Photo by John Colquhoun, DDS*) *Source*:http://www.fluoridealert.org/dental*fluorosis.htm*

Dental Fluorosis

Six types of fluorosis (Source: Fluoride Free, Ireland):

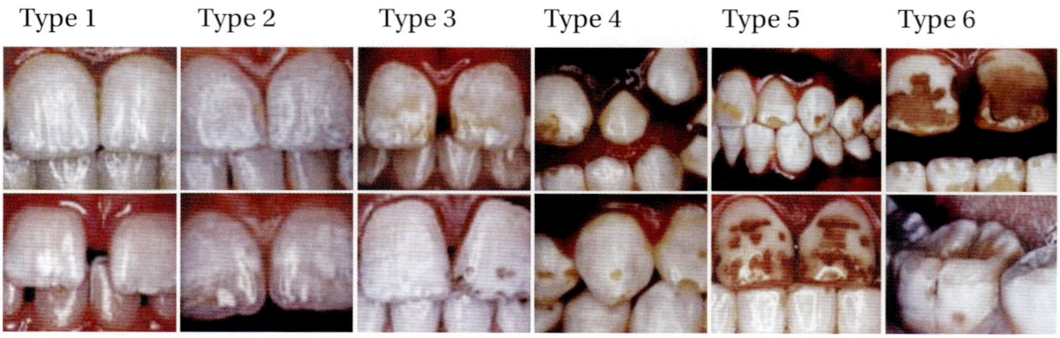

Figure 1.12: Types of fluorosis
Source: http://www.fluoridationfacts.com/education/picture%20gallery/dental_fluorosis.htm

Type 1: [Top] The earliest sign of dental fluorosis is thin white lines running across tooth. [Bottom] The tips of teeth are white and opaque.

Type 2: [Top] Unsightly white lines are more defined and are thicker. [Bottom] The tooth shows cloudy areas or thick opaque bands. Greater enamel damage.

Type 3: [Top] Brown stain superimposed on white cloudy areas. Brown stain equals enamel loss. [Bottom] Entire tooth is opaque and cloudy white. There is complete loss of translucency.

Type 4: [Top] The teeth erupt chalky white. Later the tooth displays surface damage i.e. brown discoloration. [Bottom] Further, brown pits arise due to excessive fluoride. This damage is irreversible.

Type 5: [Top] The enamel damage effects more teeth. Unsightly and weakened teeth result. [Bottom] Most of enamel has been lost from tooth surface. The protective layer is gone.

Type 6: [Top] Barely any normal enamel left. All teeth are severely effected. [Bottom] The teeth have many pits and holes. Now these teeth are more likely to decay and crumble.

Diagnosis of Dental Fluorosis from Dental Caries

- Unlike dental fluorosis, dental caries is a bacterial disorder.
- Dental caries also reveal discoloration of teeth; but unlike dental fluorosis, the discoloration in dental caries may be brown with no pattern.
- Unlike dental fluorosis, dental caries shall reveal prominent cavities visible to the naked eye.The acids produced by the bacteria shall chew up the teeth; only the stub of the teeth shall remain towards later stages.

- The cavities in dental caries shall begin between two teeth or near the base of the crown, closer to the gums where the tooth brush does not reach and food debris collects enabling the bacteria to breed and produce acids.

A typical set of teeth with dental fluorosis and dental caries are seen below:

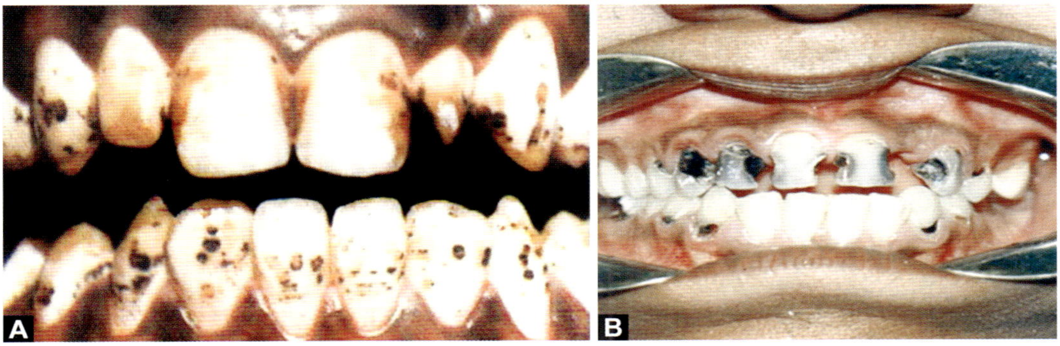

Figures 1.13A and B: (A) Dental fluorosis; (B) Dental caries

Note: Fluoride has very little role to play in rectifying cavities; except it can kill the bacteria so that no acids are formed. The same fluoride does more damage to tissue enzymes and therefore diseases surface. Using fluoride for preventing dental caries is an out dated and unethical concept.

Diagnosis of Dental Fluorosis from Dirty Teeth

- In dental fluorosis the discoloration will be on the enamel surface
- In the child shown below, the teeth of the upper jaw, the two central incisors have discoloration horizontally aligned on the enamel surface, away from the gums. It is due to dental fluorosis and is a permanent feature of the teeth
- In dirty teeth there will be discoloration of all shades but the discoloration will be along the gums (*masuda*) and not on the enamel surface.

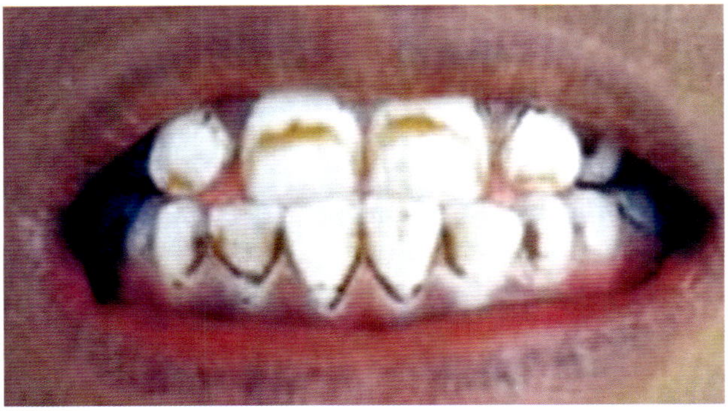

Figure 1.14: Diagnosis of dental fluorosis from dirty teeth

- The dirty teeth can be cleaned and polished by a dentist; but not in fluorosis. Whereas in the teeth of the lower jaw, there is discoloration along the gums and is due to dirty teeth, which can be cleaned by a dentist.

Skeletal Fluorosis

Skeletal fluorosis, a complicated illness caused by the accumulation of too much fluoride in the bones, has a number of stages.

The first two stages are preclinical, that is, the patient feels no symptoms but changes have taken place in the body. In the **first preclinical stage**, biochemical abnormalities occur in the blood and in bone composition; **in the second**, histological changes can be observed in the bone in biopsies. Some experts call these changes harmful because they are precursors of more serious conditions. Others say they are harmless.

In the **early clinical stage** of skeletal fluorosis, symptoms include pains in the bones and joints; sensations of burning, pricking, and tingling in the limbs; muscle weakness; chronic fatigue; and gastrointestinal disorders and reduced appetite. During this phase, changes in the pelvis and spinal column can be detected on X-rays. The bone has both a more prominent and more blurred structure.

In the **second clinical stage**, pains in the bones become constant and some of the ligaments begin to calcify. Osteoporosis may occur in the long bones, and early symptoms of osteosclerosis (a condition in which the bones become more dense and have abnormal crystalline structure) are present. Bony spurs may also appear on the limb bones, especially around the knee, the elbow and on the surface of tibia and ulna.

In **advanced skeletal fluorosis, called crippling skeletal fluorosis**, the extremities become weak and moving the joints is difficult. The vertebrae partially fuse together, crippling the patient.

Skeletal fluorosis, especially in its early stages, is a difficult disease to diagnose, and can be readily confused with various forms of arthritis including osteoarthritis and rheumatoid arthritis.

In the advanced stages, fluorosis can resemble a multitude of bone/joint diseases, including: osteosclerosis, renal osteodystrophy, DISH, spondylosis, osteomalacia, osteoporosis, and secondary hyperparathyroidism.

The risk of developing fluorosis, and the course the disease will take, is influenced by the presence of certain predisposing factors, including impaired kidney function; dietary deficiencies; gastric acidity; and repetitive stress.

"Crippling skeletal fluorosis might occur in people who have ingested 10–20 mg of fluoride per day for 10–20 years.

Skeletal fluorosis

- Vague discomfort and paresthesia in limbs and trunk are early symptoms
- Pain and stiffness in back appear later
- Stiffness increases steadily and restriction of movement occurs
- "Poker back" spine is late manifestation
- Soon stiffness spreads to various joints
- Fluorosis deformity at hips, knee and other joints are seen
- Bony exostosis seen in limb bones
- Men suffer more than women
- Skeletal fluorosis becomes crippling between 30–50 years of age in endemic areas
- New comers to endemic area develop symptoms within 4 years of arrival.

Radiological Presentations

Osteosclerosis, periosteal bone formation, calcification of interosseous membrane, ligaments, capsules, muscular attachments, tendons. Exostoses, osteophytosis, associated metabolic bone disease.

Clinical Presentation of Skeletal Fluorosis

Heel pain, painful and restricted joint movements, deformities in limbs, hunch back.

In Extreme Cases

Paralysis, muscular wasting, premature ageing.

Skeletal Fluorosis Phases

Osteosclerotic phase	*Ash concentration (mgF/kg)*	*Symptoms and signs*
Normal bone	500 to 1,000	Normal
Preclinical phase	3,500 to 5,500	Asymptomatic; slight radiographically-detectable increases in bone mass
Clinical phase I	6,000 to 7,000	Sporadic pain; stiffness of joints; osteosclerosis of pelvis and vertebral spine
Clinical phase II	7,500 to 9,000	Chronic joint pain; arthritic symptoms; slight calcification of ligaments' increased osteosclerosis and cancellous bones; with/without osteoporosis of long bones
Phase III: Crippling fluorosis	8,400	Limitation of joint movement; calcification of ligaments of neck vertebral column; crippling deformities of the spine and major joints; muscle wasting; neurological defects/ compression of spinal cord

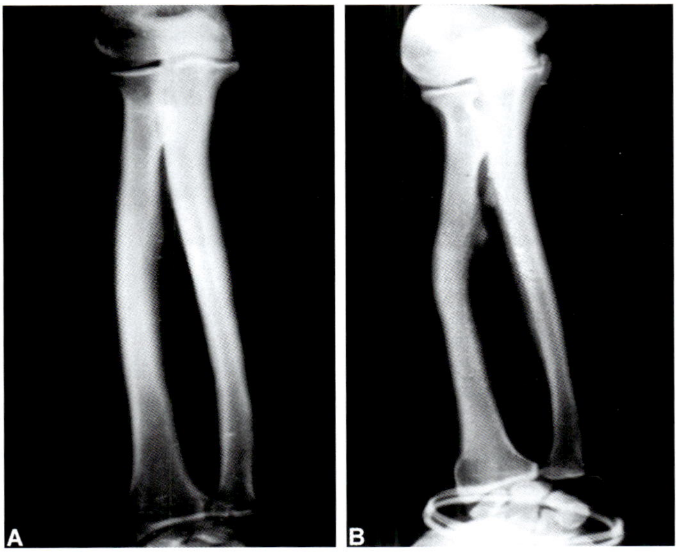

Figures 1.15A and B: (A) Normal forearm X-ray showing smooth outer and inner surfaces of the bone; (B) Forearm X-ray of a patient showing increase in bone density and calcification of the interosseous membrane

The Figure 1.15 showing increase in bone density and calcification of the interosseous membrane due to overexposure of fluoride.
Source: Journal of the International Society for Fluoride Research: http://www.fluoride-research.org/forearm/files/forearm.pdf

Non-skeletal Manifestations

Neurological manifestation: Nervousness and depression, tingling sensation in fingers and toes, excessive thirst and tendency to urinate frequently (polydypsia and plyurea): the control by brain appears to be adversely affected.

Muscular manifestations: Muscle weakness and stiffness, pain in the muscle and loss of muscle power.

Gastro - intestinal problems: Acute abdominal pain, diarrhea, constipation, blood in stool.

Edentate (Loss of teeth at an early age).

Fluoride and mental efficiency: Reduces mental work capacity (MWC) and hair zinc content.

Fluoride and thyroid: Fluoride has inhibitory effect on iodine uptake hence causing thyroid enlargement.

Fluoride and diabetes: The study showed that chronic fluoride toxicity in humans could result in significant abnormalities in glucose tolerance, which is reversible upon removal of the excess fluoride.

Non-skeletal fluorosis

- Fluoride exposure disrupts the synthesis of collagen and leads to the breakdown of collagen in bone, tendon, muscle, skin, cartilage, lungs, kidney and trachea
- Fluoride stimulates granule formation and oxygen consumption in white blood cells, but inhibits these processes when the white blood cell is challenged by a foreign agent in the blood
- Fluoride depletes the energy reserves and the ability of white blood cells to properly destroy foreign agents by the process of phagocytosis. As little as 0.2 ppm fluoride stimulates superoxide production in resting white blood cells, virtually abolishing phagocytosis. Even micro-molar amounts of fluoride, below 1 ppm, may seriously depress the ability of white blood cells to destroy pathogenic agents
- Fluoride confuses the immune system and causes it to attack the body's own tissues, and increases the tumor growth rate in cancer prone individuals
- Fluoride inhibits antibody formation in the blood
- Fluoride depresses thyroid activity
- Fluorides have a disruptive effect on various tissues in the body
- Fluoride promotes development of bone cancer
- Fluorides cause premature aging of the human body
- Fluoride ingestion from mouth rinses and dentifrices in children is extremely hazardous to biological development, life span and general health.

Fluorosis Diagnostic Tests

(For skeletal and non-skeletal fluorosis).

Fluorosis Diagnostic Tests in Adults

Tests

Fluoride to be tested in

- Drinking water (to collect in plastic bottle only)
- Blood (serum) [*fasting not required*]

- Urine (spot urine sample)
- Radiograph of the forearm
- Hemoglobin.

Fluorosis Diagnostic Tests in Children

Tests

- Fluoride in drinking water of the child; if an infant or new born, the drinking water of the mother
- Blood (serum) of the child; if an infant or new born, the blood serum of the mother
- Urine of the child/infant.

Additional Tests

- Thyroid hormone levels T3 and T4
- Thyroid stimulating hormone (TSH)
- Iodine in urine.

In Industrial Workers Fluoride to be tested in:

- Drinking water
- Blood (serum)
- Urine and urinary pH
- Nail clippings
- Hemoglobin
- Retrieval of health complaints
- Retrieval of information related to food habits.

TREATMENT AND PREVENTION: FLUORIDE AND FLUOROSIS

There is a crying need to overcome the problem of fluorosis.
Three approaches are suggested:

1. Health education
2. Treatment of the children
3. Preventive measures.

Health Education

The main area of interest will be as follows:

Creating Disease Awareness

Creating awareness about the disease should be in form of figures and presentation of the final consequences of the disease to the extent possible.

If required live presentation of the patients, who are suffering from the severe form of the disease, in areas where the gravity of problem has not reached to that extent. It may be of use, to demonstrate the most severe extent of the disease and to motivate them to use the preventive or therapeutic measures.

Creating Awareness about the Sources of the Fluoride

The creation of awareness will help in implementing the need based preventive measures in the affected community.

Community Education and Mobilization

It can be done through the booklets and several leaflets and posters (IEC materials) regarding fluorosis and its prevention.

Treatment of the Fluorosis

Treatment of fluorosis
A. Micro/macro abrasion
B. Bleaching
C. Composite restorations
D. Veneers
E. Full crowns

- Vitamins C, E and D and salts of calcium or magnesium can be used to treat chronic Fluoride toxicity.
- Antioxidants such as β-carotene, glutathione, quercetin, allicin, capasaican, ellagic acid, gallic acid, epicatechin, lycopene, glucosinolates, lutein and zeaxanthin. Antioxidants are particularly important in protecting the body from fluoride toxicity. They act as "scavengers" to remove "free radicals" and occur naturally in fresh fruit and vegetables. Vitamin E (α-tocopherol), a potent antioxidant, exerts its protective effect primarily through destruction of cell damaging free oxygen species. Vitamin C (ascorbic acid) is an antioxidant with detoxification properties. Calcium may help overcome the hypocalcemia induced by fluoride and act synergistically with vitamin C.
- The damage that dental fluorosis causes to the teeth enamel is permanent and not reversible. Dental fluorosis treatment is targeting in hiding the discoloration of the teeth.

The Treatment Options Depend on the Severity of Dental Fluorosis

Tooth Whitening: Only for Mild Fluorosis Cases

The whitening is achieved by the abrasion of the outer layer of the enamel in order to remove surface stains.

In cases of severe dental fluorosis, the tooth enamel usually becomes porous, and tooth whitening methods are not recommended as treatment. Dental fluorosis treatment for severe cases of fluorosis requires covering the affected teeth with restorations,such as :

Composite bonding: After etching the enamel, a composite resin (with a color matching the other teeth) is "glued" on to the exterior of the tooth.

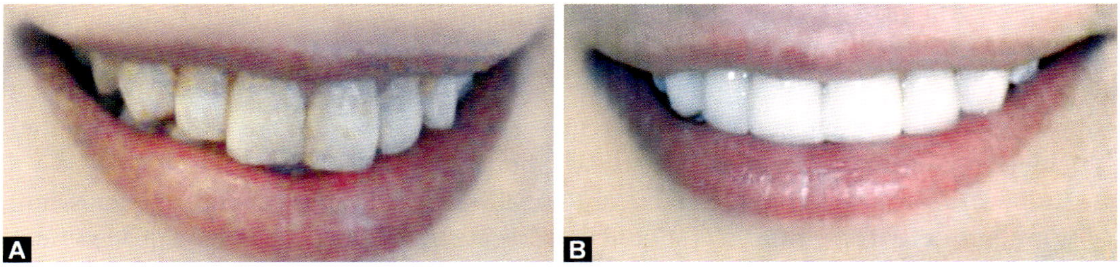

Figures 1.16A and B: (A) Fluorosis before treatment; (B) After treatment (porcelain laminate veneers)
Source: http://en.wikipedia.org/wiki/Dental_fluorosis

Porcelain veneers: Made out of porcelain, veneers form a ceramic shell over the surface of the tooth, covering the stains and discoloration caused by the dental fluorosis.

- Tooth bonding and porcelain veneers are relatively expensive dental fluorosis treatments but they can provide excellent cosmetic results.
- The presence of calcium in gut directly affects the absorption of fluoride ions and will also improve serum calcium levels as observed by Teotia, et al.
- Vitamin D3 in low doses enhances calcium absorption and retention without causing hypercalcemia and thus directly affects the absorption of fluoride ions.
- Vitamin C (ascorbic acid) controls collagen formation, maintains the teeth structure and is also essential for bone formation. These structures are adversely affected by higher fluoride intake.

Prevention

Preventing Dental Fluorosis

- Parents should take the necessary measures for preventing dental fluorosis on their children teeth
- Powdered or liquid concentrate infant formula should be mixed with water that is fluoride-free or contains low levels of fluoride
- Do not use fluoride toothpaste until the child is 2 years old unless advised to do so by a dentist
- For children age two and older, place only a pea-sized amount of fluoride toothpaste on the toothbrush at each brushing
- Avoid toothpastes with flavors that may encourage swallowing, An adult should supervise the use of fluoride-containing dental products by children younger than 6 years old, and check that they do not swallow it.

What consumer product industries and health agencies can do to reduce the occurrence of dental fluorosis?

- Label the fluoride concentration of bottled water. Producers of bottled water should label the fluoride concentration of their products. Such labeling would allow consumers to make informed decisions.

- Promote the use of a small amount of fluoride toothpaste for children younger than 6 years. Labels and advertisements for fluoride toothpaste should promote using only a pea-sized amount (0.25g) of toothpaste on a child-sized toothbrush for children younger than 6 years. Parents and caregivers should be encouraged to supervise their children's toothbrushing to reduce the swallowing of excess toothpaste.
- **Collaborate**: Professional health care organizations, public health agencies, and suppliers of oral care products should collaborate to educate health care professionals and the public.

Two alternatives have been suggested to reduce the consumption of fluoride:

- **Firstly,** a reduction in the amount of toothpaste used should be achieved by educating parents to offer small, and therefore safe, amounts of toothpaste. For children between 4 and 6 years old, parents can be taught to use an amount equivalent to "a pea size", dispending toothpaste over the toothbrush with the "transverse technique". For children in a more tender age, parents should simply touch the toothbrush inside the toothpaste cover or tube, instead of squeezing it on the toothbrush. It has to be always reminded that children under 6 years old should be monitored during tooth brushing, encouraged not to swallow toothpaste, and not to use fluoridated mouth rinses.
- The second alternative is the development of dentifrices with low fluoride concentration, which are already available in many countries.

Providing Defluoridated Water for Drinking Purpose

Desirable characteristics of defluoridation process

- Cost-effective
- Easy to handle/operate by rural population—the major sufferer
- Independent of input fluoride concentration, alkalinity, pH, temperature
- Not affect taste of water
- Not add other undesirable substances (e.g. aluminium) to treated water as it can cause toxicity.

Keeping in view the cost involved in defluoridating the water it is desirable that the defluoridation of water should be restricted to drinking water only. Hence, the only economical and practicable choice left is **Domestic Defluoridation**.

It is now desirable to test the various domestic defluoridation processes, especially in terms of acceptance by people without the need of any supervising agency, and recommend suitable alternatives so that effective long-term implementation can be achieved.

It is estimated that the daily consumption of water for all purposes per capita is about 135 lpcd in urban areas and about 40 lpcd in rural areas, whereas for drinking and food preparing purposes it is only 8 lpcd.Keeping in view the cost involved in defluoridating the water it is desirable that the defluoridation of water should be restricted to drinking water only. Hence the only economical and practicable choice left is Domestic defluoridation.

The important role of fluoride in the prevention of dental caries is evident and turns the water fluoridation into a public health measure. The fluoride level supplied in water can vary from 0.7 to 1.0 ppm, depending on the seasons of the year. Thus, as the ambient temperature gets warmer, the water intake increases, requiring lower levels of fluoride in drinking water. Fluoridated water is, directly or indirectly, responsible for 40% of dental fluorosis, through water intake or children's formula and food prepared with drinking water. The other 60% are attributed to other sources of fluoride. In a systematic review, where 214 studies were analyzed, McDonagh, et al. observed a decrease in the number of caries-affected teeth and an increase in dental fluorosis, depending on the fluoride intake. They also stated that the prevalence of dental fluorosis indicates that children are ingesting other sources of fluoride besides drinking water. In areas where drinking water is obtained directly from deep wells, dental fluorosis is often endemic and in many cases, the deeper the wells, the higher the fluoride concentration in drinking water. In order to prevent fluorosis, the pediatric dentist has to instruct parents about the fluoride content in the drinking water and when it is not known, look for this information in the local water supply service. If a child drinks well water or bottled water, the pediatric dentist may assist the parents or caregivers in getting an analysis of its fluoride content, and afterwards decide together whether the child needs a fluoride supplement or not. Dentists also should educate parents about diet, such as children's formula, food or sodas that need water to be manufactured and can indirectly participate in the development of dental fluorosis. Therefore, parents should also limit the amount of fluoride in bottled beverages.

It is now desirable to test the various domestic defluoridation processes, especially in terms of acceptance by people without the need of any supervising agency, and recommend suitable alternatives so that effective long-term implementation can be achieved.

Surprisingly none of the domestic defluoridation processes available today have been much successful in the field. Relative merits and demerits of some of these processes are as follows:

Nalgonda Process

It is a cumbersome technique not suitable for use by uneducated rural population—the section that needs it the most. Further, it is difficult to control the alum dose because it is different for each source of water. The process can be used only for water having a fluoride content of less than 10 ppm. If the alum dose is not properly controlled it may result in high residual aluminum content in output drinking water. The IS 10500 sets an absolute maximum limit of 0.2 ppm of aluminum in drinking water. Excess of alum also renders metallic taste to the water.

Activated Alumina Process

It is an expensive process. Reactivation of filter material is cumbersome and it can be done only with the help of trained persons generally not available in most of our villages. This process also results in high residual aluminum in output water ranging from 0.16 ppm to 0.45 ppm.

Other Processes

Processes like electrodialysis, reverse osmosis, etc. require special equipment, electrical energy and especially trained persons to operate these units. Operation and maintenance of these units is also very expensive and hence these are not suitable as domestic defluoridation processes for use in rural areas.

Recently KRASS have come out with new defluoridation process named **KDP** (**KRASS defluoridation process)**, which have shown promising results.

The salient features are given below:

In this process the fluoride contaminated water passed through the bed of media by any means such as filter to get the defluoridated water. This process differs from the known processes in its simplicity, cost effectiveness and **very low traces of residual aluminum** in outlet water. There is no limit on fluoride concentration in input water. Temperature, pH, alkalinity and total dissolved solids of input water do not affect this process. The ambient conditions like atmospheric temperature and humidity do not have any effect on this process. It is a practical approach especially for our rural population.

The importance of the process is a defluoridation process, which is easy, to use by illiterate villagers, requires minimal involvement of technical personnel, is harmless and is cost-effective. In the process, once the filter are laid at a door step, the inflow of the fluoride rich water is without further expenditure in terms of cost except recharging according to the capacity of filter. The exhausted media bed can be easily recharged again without replacing the material at least upto 40 cycles. As a product, the process achieves better removal of suspended matter, betters clarity and maintains taste of water. The treatment cost is about 0.6–0.8 paisa per liter at 10 ppm of influent fluoride.

Changing the Dietary Habits

Deflouridation of drinking water alone shall not bring the fluoride level to a safe limit. It would be necessary to overcome the toxic effects of the remaining fluoride ingested through other source. This can be done by effecting minor changes in the diet and dietary habits of the population compatible with their social system and available resources. The main aim should be to:

- Restrict use of fluoride rich food
- Avoiding use of fluoride rich toothpastes
- Use of food rich in calcium, vitamin C and proteins like *Amla, Shalgam ka sag, Hara dhania, Ajwayan, Til,* skimmed milk powder, etc.

The clinicians must be aware of the optimum concentration of fluoride needed in water, before prescribing them. Fluorosis can be prevented if pediatricians, as well as dentists, follow the new guidelines for fluoride supplements, and be aware that these supplements are not recommended for children who are exposed to water supplies with an adequate amount of fluoride.

Fluorosis can be prevented by monitoring the amount of fluoride that children up to 6 years old are exposed, therefore, the dentist must be aware of the main sources of fluoride to prevent fluorosis and instruct parents or caregivers on how daily dose should be managed in order to achieve success in prevention.

The excessive fluoride intake, in consequence to the inadequate use or swallowing of fluoride-containing toothpastes, is also responsible for the development of dental fluorosis. Children up to 5 years old swallow around 30% of the amount of toothpaste used every time they brush their teeth. If fluoridated water is consumed at the same time, a potential risk of dental fluorosis occurs.

Water Harvesting (Alternative Water Source)

Fluoride not only affects the people but it also affects the animals. The water harvesting technologies should be aimed not only to provide fluoride-free water to human beings but also to animals. Rainwater storage can be a major source of fluoride-free drinking water for the animals.

This three pronged attack can prove to be a blessing for the population especially for the younger generation living in fluoride rich areas having no choice except to drink the water contaminated with fluoride and suffer the inevitable consequences including permanent deformities.

BENEFITS

From this research study the people of North Gujarat who are already afflicted with fluorosis will be benefitted .This study aims to bring a close insight into the gravity of the fluorosis problem and the causative factors responsible for it. It will also assess the effect of mitigation measures undertaken to alleviate fluorosis like Dharoi water supply and subsequently what is needed further.

RATIONALE

"Fluoride is a worldwide menace" as Fred Pearce expressed in his article **(www.fluoride.org.uk/news/news_index.htm).**

Fluorosis doesn't cause any severe mortality and morbidity but it can make the person cripple which is more deplorable rather than being dead. There is decrease in working efficiency of the people because of joint and back pain.These people become burden to society and their families as there is decrease in working capacity, earnings and self confidence. Another social aspect of the problem is that young girls have difficulty in marriages because of discoloration of teeth.

There is paucity of information and scientific study on fluorosis. This study has been undertaken to have a deeper insight in comprehending the fluorosis condition in endemic areas of North Gujarat. This study also aims to throw light on the impact of mitigation measures taken to curb fluorosis in North Gujarat like water supply from Dharoi dam. The perception and knowledge of the people regarding water quality and fluorosis has also been taken into account to capture overall impact of fluorosis on society.

There have been no comprehensive health surveys for dental fluorosis from which the overall extent of the problem could be assessed. The dental fluorosis has been captured deeply in this study in endemic areas of North Gujarat based on Deans Fluorosis Indices. The thing which is most peculiar in this study is that DF not always means discolored tooth but also white opacities which can be classified into mild DF and this issue has been taken into consideration in this study.

Overall the effort has been made to capture physical, social, economical and cultural aspects of fluorosis on society. A comparison has also been made with previous studies on fluorosis which were done in same villages of North Gujarat by studying the same families as it was done in the following survey (Shah and Indu).

2

AIMS AND OBJECTIVES

AIM

To do a trend analysis of fluorosis in North Gujarat.

OBJECTIVES

- To assess the prevalence and severity of dental and skeletal fluorosis in the endemic areas of North Gujarat
- To assess the categories/grades of the dental fluorosis in segment of the population based on fluorosis indices
- To assess the impact of fluorosis mitigation measures like water supply from Dharoi dam, in endemic areas of North Gujarat by making a primarily qualitative comparison of individual physical symptoms between pre and post-implementation (of mitigation measures) phase
- To study the awareness about fluorosis and perception of the quality of water among people.

3

LITERATURE REIVEW

There are lots of communicable diseases like T.B., malaria, HIV, measles, polio, etc. for which majority of national programs are going on. There are also some non-communicable diseases, which are of public health importance like cardiovascular and respiratory diseases, diabetes, cancers, etc. **Fluorosis is also a non-communicable disease with estimate of 65 million people affected as cited by Dr Susheela, A K.** Severe skeletal fluorosis can make a person cripple and unproductive, results in huge economic burden and thus it fits to be qualified as a major public health problem. Following literature were studied for this study on fluorosis:

REVERSAL OF FLUOROSIS IN CHILDREN

S K Gupta, R C Gupta, A K Seth and A Gupta Jaipur, India
Abstract from Acta Paediatrica Japonica 38 (5) 513–19, 1996 (http://www.ncbi.nlm.nih.gov/pubmed/8942013)

This paper stresses the role of nutrients, i.e. calcium, vit. C and vit. D for the treatment of fluorosis. Large population consumes fluoride-contaminated water, especially in developing countries. The toxic effects of fluorosis take three forms: clinical, skeletal and dental. Research thus far indicates that the manifestations of fluorosis are irreversible. However, it has been observed that the ingestion of calcium, vitamin C or vitamin D, individually, is effective in protection from fluoride toxicity to a certain extent. Therefore, a double blind control trial was conducted to examine the effect of a combination of calcium, vitamin D, and ascorbic acid supplementation in fluorosis-affected children. The children were given ascorbic acid, calcium and vitamin D, well below the toxic dosages in a double blind manner using lactose as a placebo. Follow up revealed a significant improvement in dental, clinical and skeletal fluorosis and relevant biochemical parameters in these children. Thus, the study indicated that fluorosis can be reversed, at least in children, by a therapeutic regimen that is fairly cheap, simple and easily available and without any side effects.

THE FLUORIDE DEBATE: A RESPONSE TO AMERICAN DENTAL ASSOCIATIONS BOOKLET, FLUORIDATION FACTS

National survey of U.S. school children conducted by the National Institute of Dental Research, 1986-87 (http://www.fluoridedebate.com/question19.html)

In this survey, dental fluorosis has been classified using Dean's Fluorosis Index, the tooth present in an individual's mouth is rated according to the fluorosis index. The individual's Fluorosis score is based upon the severest form of fluorosis recorded for two or more teeth.

In this dental fluorosis was present in 22.3% of the children examined using Dean's Index. These children were exposed to all sources of fluoride (fluoridated water, food, beverages, fluoride dental products and dietary supplements). The prevalence of the types of fluorosis was:

- Very mild fluorosis 17.0%
- Mild fluorosis 4.0%
- Moderate fluorosis 1.0%
- Severe fluorosis 0.3%
- Total cases of fluorosis 22.3%.

The incidence of moderate or severe fluorosis comprised a very small portion (6%) of the total amount of fluorosis. In other words, 94% of all dental fluorosis is the very mild to mild form of dental fluorosis.

FLUOROSIS IN GUJARAT: A DISASTER AHEAD

By Tushaar Shah and Rajnarayan Indu IWMI Study 2004 (http://www.carewater.org/fluorosisNG.pdf)

In this study, the prevalence of fluorosis was studied in 25 villages, by taking a census survey using a short questionnaire.

In this study, about six very visible symptoms of Fluorosis were inquired in the census questionnaire.

Besides person-wise family details, the information was collected about whether a person is affected by any of the following symptoms related to fluorosis:

1. Dental fluorosis
2. Can touch chest with chin
3. Can bend forward easily
4. Can do sit-ups
5. Can touch back of the head with hands
6. Crippled.

Dental fluorosis has been placed separately.A person is called 'afflicted' with Fluorosis or MSD, when one gives a negative reply totat least one of the (2) to (6) symptoms. Then the percent of afflicted persons over the total population was calculated as the 'prevalence' rate of fluorosis or MSD in the 25 villages. Out of 28,425 people examined in 25 villages nearly 36% or 10,126 persons were suffering from dental fluorosis (DF) and 16% or 4,590 persons were suffering from at least one of the five symptoms of Fluorosis. Among 4590 affected persons, 14% or 643 cannot even walk properly and more than 64% cannot sit up and bend forward properly in Gujarat.The samples of water were collected from the different sources in the 25 villages used for drinking and were tested for their TDS and fluoride content in the laboratory. The content of fluoride and TDS were found to be source specific.

MEHSANA FLUORIDE AREA HEALTH BASELINE SURVEY

By Desai, Dr (Mrs) Vikas K; Govt.Medical College, Surat 1993. (http://www.carewater.org/fluorosisNG.pdf)

The 25 villages were surveyed by the team headed by Dr (Mrs) Vikas Desai .This Project was surveyed in 1993 and the report was brought out in 1994 under the name of 'Mehsana Fluoride Area Health Baseline Survey'.

With a team of doctors, she did a baseline survey in and around Mehsana. This study has primarily focused on preparing the baseline of sanitation, health, nutrition, and fluorosis problem for future impact assessment. In this study the prevalence rate of skeletal fluorosis, non-skeletal fluorosis and dental fluorosis were studied separately.

UNDERSTANDING THE DISEASE OF ENDEMIC SKELETAL FLUOROSIS AND WAYS TO CONTAIN IT

By D Raja Reddy
(http://www.fluorosisinandhra.org/Booklet_Fluorosis.pdf)

This study was based in the villages of Andhra Pradesh.

In this study, the three factors were identified for the causation of skeletal fluorosis, i.e. water, food and nutrition. It stresses the use of Krishna water for drinking and cooking for every fluorotic village and trying it for cultivation in future. It also emphasizes improving the nutrition of the population especially those of growing children by whatever means practicable. Avoiding drinks such as tea, which is very rich in fluoride and also sea foods. Avoiding analgesics, which could damage the kidneys and aggravate the problem in these areas where studies reveal a higher incidence of kidney disease.

ENDEMIC FLUOROSIS IN SOUTHERN RAJASTHAN

By SL Choubisa Dungarpur, Rajasthan, India, Fluoride Vol. 34 No. 1 61-70 2001 Research Report 61
(http://www.fluoride-journal.com/01-34-1/341-61.pdf)

In this study, chronic fluoride intoxication in the form of osteo-dental fluorosis was investigated in 21 villages of Banswara, Dungarpur, and Udaipur district of southern Rajasthan, where fluoride (F) concentrations in drinking waters range from 1.5 to 4.0 ppm.

A cross-sectional survey was used to determine the prevalence of fluorosis. Teeth of children and adults of both sexes were examined for evidence of dental fluorosis, using grade II mottling as a criterion. For skeletal fluorosis, adults over the age of 21 who had lived in one of the villages for more than 15 years were included in the study and were examined clinically as described elsewhere.

At 1.5 ppm, 21.3, 25.6 and 38.9% of children and 33.3, 36.9 and 44.8% of adults in different villages of these districts were found to be affected with dental fluorosis. The maximum prevalence of dental fluorosis (77.1%) was found in the 17–22 years age group.

At this 1.5 ppm fluoride concentration, 6.1, 6.8 and 9.5% of adults in villages of Banswara, Udaipur, and Dungarpur districts, respectively, showed evidence of skeletal fluorosis. Subjects of these districts showed the highest prevalence of skeletal fluorosis, 32.8, 36.6, and 39.2% at maximum fluoride level of 3.7 ppm, 4.0 ppm and 3.2 ppm, respectively.

4

METHODOLOGY

The villages of North Gujarat have been selected for this survey to have more accurate and deeper insight into the gravity of the Fluorosis problem due to following reason.

There is a high demand for groundwater for domestic use. However, deepening wells to harvest groundwater unmindfully, deepens the problem of contamination with fluoride, nitrate, arsenic etc; especially, when it is extracted from underground, where water sits in pores in the rocks for long periods like in Aravalli Range in North Gujarat. Escalating water crisis in North Gujarat forces people to search for water deeper and deeper underground that has aggravated the problem of fluoride contamination. The problem becomes more acute when rainfall is less (**Shah and Indu**).

Background of Mehsana District

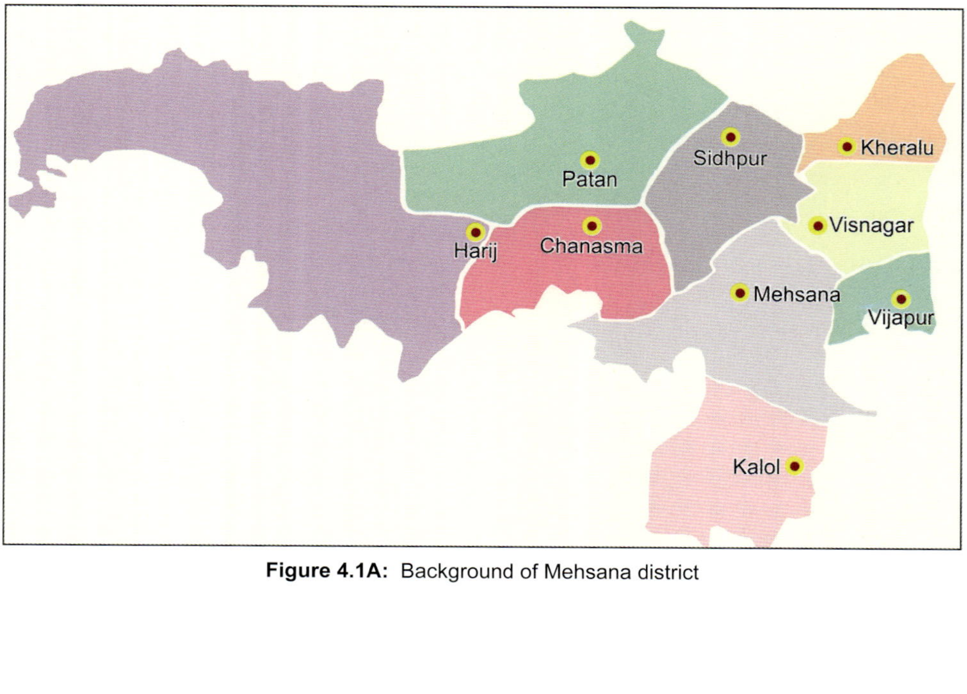

Figure 4.1A: Background of Mehsana district

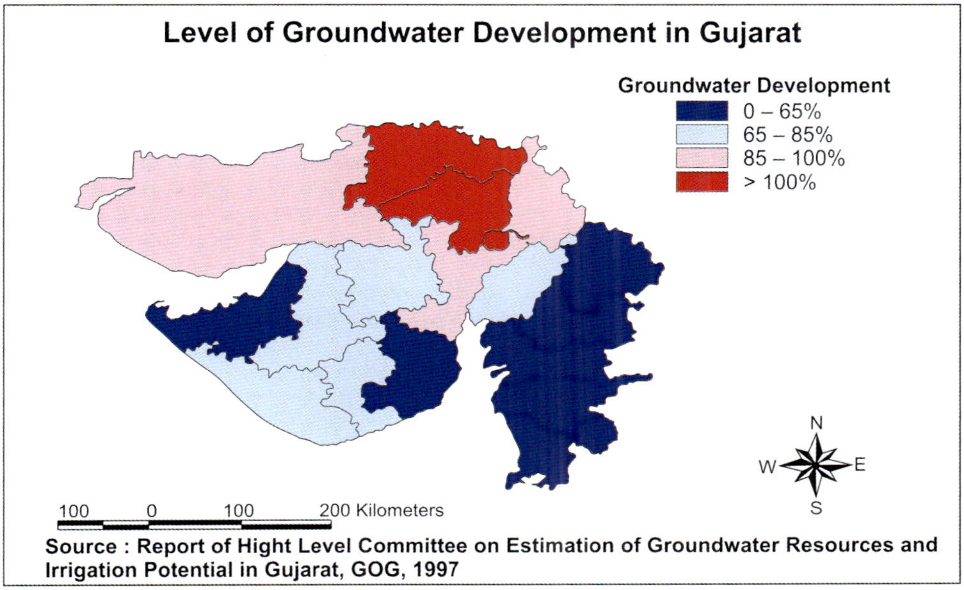

Figure 4.1B: Level of groundwater development in Gujarat
Source: Mehsana district profile booklet, 2006-07

Introduction: Mehsana

Mehsana districtis located in North Gujarat, about 75 km from Ahmedabad .The district borders with Banaskantha district in the north, Patan and Surendranagar districts in the west, Gandhinagar and Ahmedabad districts in the south and Sabarkantha district in the east.The major crops of mehsana are potato, cotton, tobacco, oilseeds, castor seeds, cumin, psyllium and anise.

Asia's second largest dairy 'Dudhsagar Milk Cooperative Dairy'and largest market yard 'Unjha' is located in Mehsana.'Sun Temple' at Modhera is an important tourist destination of Mehsana district.

Nine Talukas of Mehsana district are:

1. Satlasana
2. Kheralu
3. Unjha
4. Vadnagar
5. Visnagar
6. Becharaji
7. Mehsana
8. Vijapur
9. Kadi

Background of Patan District

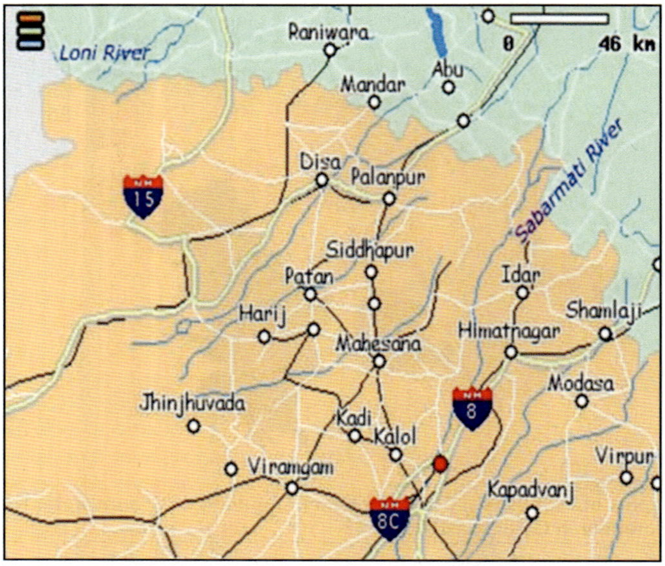

Figure 4.2: Background of Patan district

Introduction: Patan

Patan district was formed on 2-10-97 from the parts of Mehsana and Banaskantha Districts. Patan district was formed including Patan, Siddhapur, Chanasma, Harij and Sami talukas of Mahesana district and Radhanpur and Santalpur talukas of Banaskantha district. The head quarter of the district is Patan.

Seven Talukas of Patan District are:

1. Patan
2. Siddhpur
3. Chanasma
4. Harij
5. Sami
6. Radhanpur
7. Sakul

Patan District is situated between 20° 41' to 23° 55' north latitudes and east longitude of 71° 31' to 72° 20'. The area of Patan district is 5600 sq km. In the north and north-west borders, there is Banaskantha district and in the west there is the border of Kutch district. In the south and south-east there is desert of Kutch and some part of Surendranagar district. Besides this, there is Mehsana district situated in the east part of Patan.

The important tourist places in Patan district are Rankivav, Sahastraleeng lake and Rudra Mahalay. Patan is also famous for its Patola sarees.

Study Design: Population based survey.

Duration of study: From 1 April to 30 June.

Study Area: Ten fluorosis endemic villages of Mehsana and Patan districts.

Study Tools: Population sample survey was done using a short semi-structured questionnaire.

Sampling Technique

Considering the limited time available for this study, the 10 villages were selected out of the same 25 villages, which were surveyed by the team headed by Dr Rajnarayan Indu and Dr Tushaar Shah in 2004. This project was surveyed as **IWMI's** Study in 2004 under the name of "**Fluorosis in Gujarat: A Disaster Ahead**"

Selection of Ten Villages

The present prevalence rate of fluorosis was determined in the 10 villages for the seven years space, by taking a population based census survey using a short questionnaire. This census survey was done by taking following steps:

- The detailed information was collected from 100 households in 10 out of the 25 census villages of North Gujarat through a semi structured questionnaire.
- Each one of 25 villages were arranged according to Average Fluoride levels in ppm of **IWMI's Study (2004)** in a descending order. Out of this six villages were selected having fluoride levels above 4 ppm and four villages were selected having fluoride levels below 2 ppm in a randomized manner for the effective comparison of the Fluorosis afflicted persons using water having more and less fluoride levels as shown in the Table 4.1.

Table 4.1: Average water fluoride levels of the 10 villages in ppm in IWMI study

Village	*Average water fluoride in ppm in IWMI study*
Sojintra	6.5
Karsanpura	6.1
Ruppur	6
Rajgarh	5.6
Machhava	5.6
Hansapur	4.1
Karanpur	1.89
Mudana	1.28
Surpura	1.01
Pachakwada	0.99

- Once the villages were selected, the same families who were surveyed in 2004 were listed out. Following this, the families were stratified as per the present severity of problem in family members.Only those families were selected which were having more severity of the problems like joint or backache or Va.Out of such families, ten were finally selected randomly for the study.

- The six very visible symptoms of fluorosis were inquired in the census questionnaire: Besides person-wise family details, the following information was collected like whether a person is affected by any of the following symptoms related to fluorosis :
  1. Dental fluorosis
  2. Can touch chest with chin
  3. Can bend forward easily
  4. Can do sit-ups
  5. Can touch back of the head with hands
  6. Crippled.

A person is called 'afflicted' with fluorosis or MSD, when one gives a negative reply to at least one of the (2) to (6) symptoms. Then the 'prevalence' rate of fluorosis or MSD in the 10 villages was determined by dividing the total no. of afflicted persons over the total number of persons in percentage. This is a very simple estimate, since other clinical symptoms related to fluorosis were not considered and no urine and blood samples were taken for fluoride examination.

The non-skeletal fluorosis was also captured in this census survey by questioning the gastric trouble symptoms (early warning signals of fluorosis).

The dental fluorosis has been studied separately based on Deans Fluorosis Index. In 1934, Dean developed a classification for fluorosis, which is still widely used, based on his interpretation of clinical appearance. Dean and Mckay suggested that optimum level of water fluoride should be below 0.9–1.0 ppm.The dental fluorosis was classified into mild, moderate and severe based on Dean's Index criteria. Then the prevalence of dental fluorosis was determined by dividing the afflicted persons having DF with the total number of persons examined in percentage.

Dental fluorosis is visible only in children in the permanent teeth as permanent tooth starts erupting at the age of 6 years and the discoloration and white opacities are clearly visible with naked eye but it requires specialist dental examination.

Ethical Clearance and Informed Consent

Before starting the study, ethical clearance was obtained from the Ethical Committee of Indian Institute of Public Health, Gandhinagar. Verbal with written consent was obtained from the respondents of the families before commencement of the study as there were no invasive procedures or drug intervention in the study.

The identities of the respondents were kept confidential during the study period and also during analysis and after publication of the study.

5

INFERENCES

FIELD VISIT EXPERIENCE

Vital excerpts of the field study—from 5 May to 15 May 2010:

It was very startling yet a prolific experience of mine first field visit as a public health person. The hundred families in ten villages of Mehsana and Patan districts of North Gujarat were surveyed in this census survey. Whatever being read about fluorosis condition in papers, books, net, case studies, journals, etc. that was live in front of us. Ours mind started comparing the theoretical context of deplorable fluorosis condition with live aggrieved and afflicted people in these villages.

The eyes of the afflicted people gave the impression of blending of sorrow and faint hope. To get good quality of water is like a distant dream for them. Dharoi water supply seems to be like a mirage for them. The people of all the villages were very cooperative and heartily cooperated us in this study with a ray of hope in their eyes regarding regular and qualitative water supply.

Around 60% of families receive Dharoi water and 40% of families still don't receive Dharoi water supply which was initiated as one of the Govt. project to mitigate the effect of fluorosis condition and to supply safe and quality drinking water to the people of the villages of North Gujarat. Those who are receiving still don't have regular supply and to meet their demands they are forced to mix Dharoi water with borewell water as said by one of the family person.

In one of the family visited, it was a very pitiable condition. The financial condition was very poor and both husband and wife were suffering from skeletal fluorosis. Their earning and working capacity was drastically reduced because of pain and difficulty in walking.

There was one family in which the person was bedridden/crippled and couldn't do any work. His house was tattered and he was forced to give his land under private hands for the farming. He was suffering from severe skeletal fluorosis since a long time and other persons had to escort and accompany him for the doctors visit. He had spent lots of money for this without any relief. In one of the educated family the respondent was a teacher. His wife was seriously afflicted with joint and back pain. He has spent lakhs of rupees for the treatment without any relief. He strongly urged for the quality water supply.

Another one pitiable instance was that one of the person of the village who helped us in getting touch with the affected families himself was suffering from severe skeletal fluorosis. He was not able to walk properly still he helped us inspite of our frequent refusal. He wanted to alleviate the false impression of the Government about the safe and quality water supply. He also photographed himself quiet willingly to show it to the government that the people in whole villages are suffering from pain which has made their lives miserable.

In one of the family, the fluorosis afflicted person told that the joint and back pain is the story of each house in the village. One of the person in the village was very much concerned about the discoloration of teeth of his children that he has vowed not to use borewell water for drinking purpose. He told that he will work hard to earn money for purchasing RO water for the better future of their children.He and his wife has discolored teeth and he knew that it's because of salted water. One of the family person revealed us a pot having granular salt quiet anxiously and overtly to make us clear that they are forced to drink such water as there is no other option available.

In India, a village person has to fight hard to earn bread and butter but after visiting these villages, I must say that they are yelling and striving hard to get good quality water. The bad quality water has made them crippled and has drastically reduced their earning capacity and efficiency.

OBSERVATIONS, ANALYSIS AND DISCUSSION

All above mentioned field experience has been proved by the following observations and data analysis.

Demography

In this census survey, hundred families were examined in ten villages with total of 473 members.

- Total families examined=100
- Total no. of male =250
- Total no. of females =223
- Total family members = 473

Education

Majority of people are Non SSC and SSC-HSC as shown in Table 5.1

Table 5.1: Study of education variation among people

Education	NA<5 years	Not at all	Non SSC	SSS-HSC	Graduate	PG	Others	Total
No. of persons (%)	26 (5.5)	53 (11.2)	240 (50.7)	121 (25.6)	20 (4.2)	11 (2.3)	2 (0.4)	473

Occupation

Out of 100 families 68 are engaged in farming, 14 are in service/teacher, 5 are in business and 12 are in others as shown in Table 5.2. Majority of families are engaged in farming. One family has both service/teacher and farming as their business.

Table 5.2: Study of occupation variation among people

Occupation	Farming	Service/teacher	Business	Others	Both	Total
No. of families (%)	68 (68)	14 (14)	5 (5)	12 (12)	1(1)	100

Water Supply

Out of 100 families, 61 families receive water from Dharoi and 39 families don't receive Dharoi water supply. Dharoi water supply was introduced for the villages of North Gujarat as the most sought after initiative to provide good quality water with less fluoride levels to curb the menace of fluorosis.

Around 60% of families receive Dharoi water and 40% of families still don't receive Dharoi water as shown in Table 5.3. Incidentally those who are receiving still don't have regular supply and to meet their demands they are forced to mix Dharoi water with borewell water as said by one of the family person. They are forced to deepen the borewell to meet their demands. More the deepening, more will be the fluoride level.There are also other problems for irregular supply like pipeline leakage or lack of pressure or hefty bill payments to get Dharoi water. There were certain misconceptions linked to the non-utilization of Dharoi water like water is very cold and filthy and dirty. Some families said that it causes cough and has foul odor and taste. All these factors potentiate the inadequate utilization of Dharoi water having less fluoride level.People store water daily.The distance of source of water utilized by the people in these villages varies from half to one kilometer.

Table 5.3: Study of families in terms of distribution according to availability of Dharoi water supply

Water supply	Dharoi water supply	No Dharoi water supply
No. of families	61	39

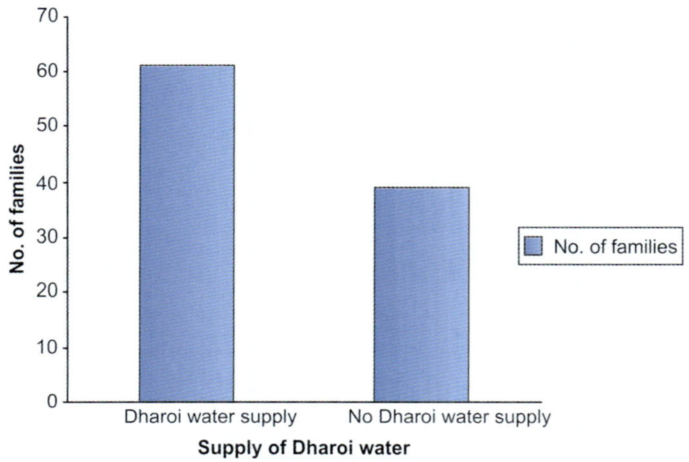

Figure 5.1: Study of families in terms of distribution as per accessibility to Dharoi water supply

Duration of Dharoi Water Supply

This observation reveals irregular supply of Dharoi water as shown in Table 5.4.

Table 5.4: Study of families in terms of duration of Dharoi water supply

Duration of Dharoi water supply in years	Total no. of families receiving Dharoi water supply	No. of families	Duration of Dharoi water supply [days per month (d/m) and hours per day (h/d)]
From last 4 years	10	10	30d/m and 4h/d
From last 6 years	30	10	20d/m and 2h/d
		10	20d/m and 4h/d
		10	30d/m and 4h/d
From last 8 years	21	10	28d/m and 2h/d
		11	30d/m and 4h/d

Perception of Dharoi Water Quality Among the Families

Out of 61 families, 6 families say that Dharoi water is of bad quality as shown in Table 5.4.

Table 5.5: Study of families in terms of perception of Dharoi water quality

Dharoi water	Good quality	Bad quality
No. of families	55	6

Distribution of Dharoi Water used for Drinking and Cooking Purpose

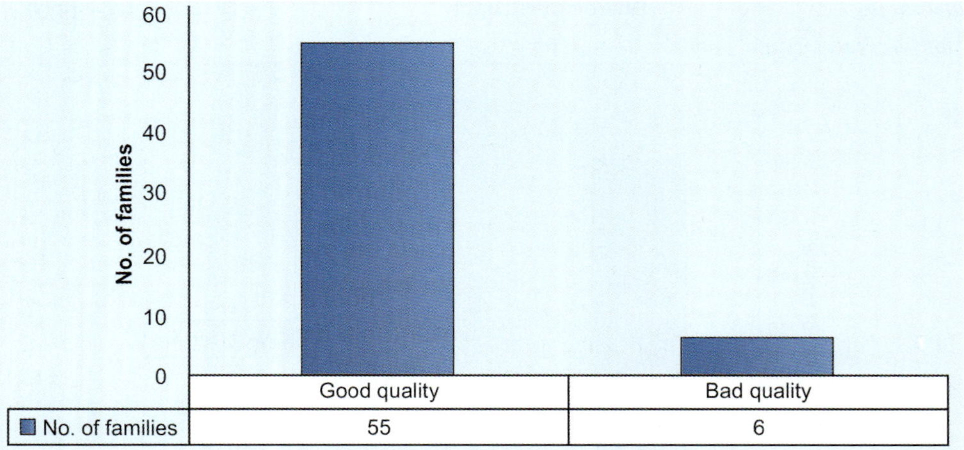

Figure 5.2: Study of families in terms of perception of Dhraoi water quality

Around 82% of the families are using only 50% of the daily usage of Dharoi water for drinking and cooking as shown in Table 5.6. None of the family is using 100% of Dharoi water for drinking and cooking which itself potentiate the fact of the grim condition of fluorosis.

Table 5.6: Study of families in terms of distribution according to use of Dharoi water

Percentage of Dharoi water used for drinking and cooking	*No. of families*
0–25%	25
25–50%	25
50–75%	11
75–100%	0

Perception of Pain with duration of Dharoi Water Supply

Out of 100 families, majority of the families were of the view that there is no relief in pain at all after using Dharoi water as shown in Tables 5.7 to 5.9. The duration of Dharoi water supply is not regular and on top of it majority of families are using only 50% of Dharoi water for drinking and cooking purposes. The people also have certain misconceptions about non-usage of Dharoi water. All these factors support the above mentioned fact of non-relief in the joint and back pain.

Table 5.7: Perception of joint and back pain after supply of Dharoi water

Symptoms	*Remained same (No. of families) (%)*	*Decreased (No. of families) (%)*	*Increased (No. of families) (%)*	*Not replied (No. of families) (%)*	*Total HHs*
Joint pain	42 (70)	12 (20)	6 (10)	40 (40)	100
Back pain	32 (66.7)	10 (20.8)	6 (12.5)	52 (52)	100

Table 5.8: Perception of joint pain with duration of the supply of Dharoi water

Duration of Dharoi water supply	*Joint pain (No. of families) (%)*		
	Remained same	*Decreased*	*Increased*
4	8 (88.9)	1 (11.1)	0 (0)
6	20 (66.7)	8 (26.7)	2 (6.7)
8	14 (66.7)	3 (14.3)	4 (19)

Table 5.9: Perception of back pain with duration of the supply of Dharoi water

Duration of Dharoi water supply (years)	*Back pain (No. of families) (%)*		
	Remained same	*Decreased*	*Increased*
4	3 (100)	0 (0)	0 (0)
6	18 (66.7)	7 (25.9)	2 (7.4)
8	13 (65)	3 (15)	4 (20)

The Prevalence of DF and Musculoskeletal Fluorosis

The five symptoms which have been taken for this survey are the basic physical symptoms of 'fluorosis' to be checked initially for diagnosing fluorosis' (Susheela, 2001, 48). In an endemic locale, where water is contaminated with excess fluoride and is being used by the local population for a long time, and also if any of these five symptoms are found in a person, then that person should be taken for further investigation for 'fluorosis'. It's wondering that whether these affected persons can be termed as 'fluorosis-prone' people. In that case, instead of putting them under the heading of MSD, they are kept under 'fluorosis-afflicted' people. Therefore, now onwards all MSD or 'Va' cases shall be referred as 'fluorosis-afflicted' or simply refer as 'fluorosis' cases.

Dental Fluorosis

In 100 families, 'having 473 family members around 282 persons were examined clinically for dental fluorosis. Out of 282 persons, according to DEAN's fluorosis criteria, mild fluorosis was present in 125 persons, moderate fluorosis in 72 persons, severe fluorosis in 12 persons, fluorosis absent in 36 persons and 37 people were not identified because they were edentulous or partially edentulous as shown in Table 5.10. This criteria for classification of dental fluorosis is different than that used in IWMI's study (2004).

Mild fluorosis was present in maximum number of persons that is almost 44.3% which is quite significant. **"Dean advised that when the average child in a community has mild Fluorosis,". . . it begins to constitute a public health problem warranting increasing consideration" (Dean 1942, p. 29)." NRC 2006 p 106.**

The prevalence of dental fluorosis is 74.1% among 282 people examined.

Table 5.10: Classification of dental fluorosis based on Dean's Index Criteria

Dental fluorosis	*No. of persons (total 282)*	*Percentage of persons*
Mild fluorosis	125	44.3
Moderate fluorosis	72	25.5
Severe fluorosis	12	4.3
Absent	36	12.8
NA	37	13.1

Village Wise Distribution of DF

Majority of the villages have more than 70% of people suffering from Dental Fluorosis out of 282 persons examined according to Deans Index Criteria as shown in following Tables 5.11 and 5.12.

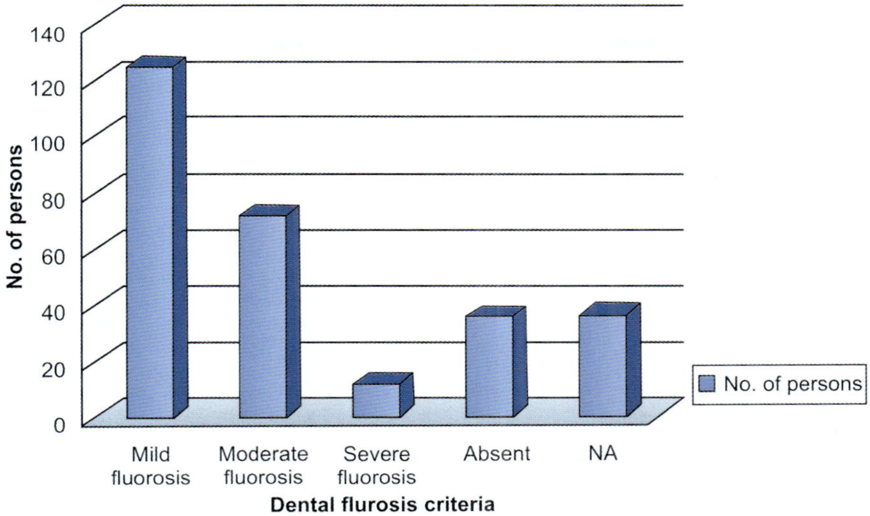

Figure 5.3: Classification of DF based on Dean's Index Criteria

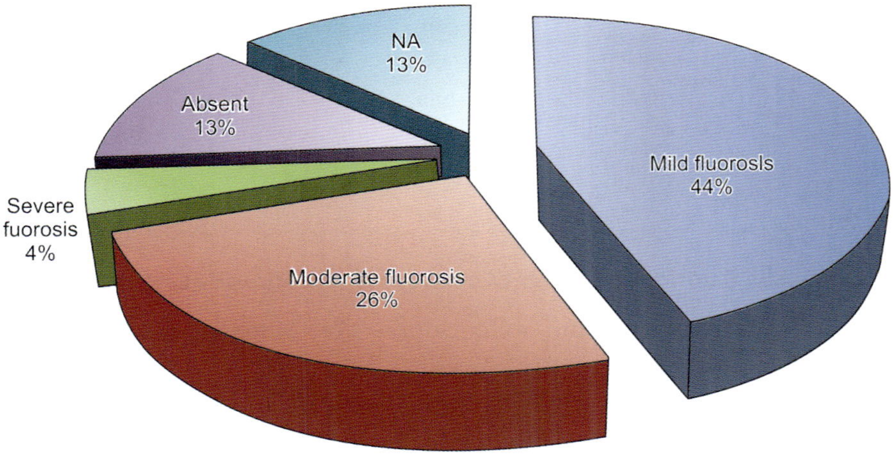

Figure 5.4: Grades of DF based on Dean's Index Criteria

Table 5.11: Study of villages in terms of prevalence of dental fluorosis

Villages	*Total no. of persons examined (282)*	*Stages of fluorosis*					*Total No. of fluorosis pt. (209)*	*Percentage of DF*
		Mild	*Moderate*	*Severe*	*Absent*	*NA*		
Karanpur	24	14	2	1	4	3	17	70.8
Surpura	25	16	3	0	5	1	19	76.0
Rajgarh	31	12	11	0	2	6	23	74.2
Karsanpura	29	14	7	1	0	7	22	75.9
Machava	35	16	5	2	7	5	23	65.7
Hansapur	31	6	21	3	1	0	30	96.8
Pachakvada	29	20	3	0	5	1	23	79.3
Mudana	27	12	6	0	7	2	18	66.7
Ruppur	24	7	6	0	3	8	13	54.2
Sojintra	27	8	8	5	2	4	21	77.8

Table 5.12: Study of villages in terms of prevalence of DF in relation to average water fluoride levels

Village	*Average water fluoride in IWMI study*	*Percentage of DF*
Sojintra	6.5	77.8
Karsanpura	6.1	75.9
Ruppur	6	54.2
Rajgarh	5.6	74.2
Machhava	5.6	65.7
Hansapur	4.1	96.8
Karanpur	1.89	70.8
Mudana	1.28	66.7
Surpura	1.01	76
Pachakwada	0.99	79.3

Dental Fluorosis in Relation to Dharoi Water Supply and Fluoride Levels

The villages which receive dharoi water supply are: Mudana, Pachakvada, Surpura, Karanpur, Macchava and Karsanpura.

The villages which don't receive Dharoi water supply are: Rajgarh, Hansapur, Ruppur and Sojintra.

This observation reveals that the villages having more fluoride levels have greater number of cases of dental fluorosis.

If we compare dental fluorosis with availability and non-availability of Dharoi water then in both of the cases more than 70% of the people shows the symptoms of dental fluorosis according to Deans Index Criteria as shown in Tables 5.13 and 5.14. The slight difference observed can be attributed to higher fluoride levels in the villages without Dharoi water supply.

By surprise it was observed that those villages having more fluoride levels have no supply of Dharoi water. Those villages which receive Dharoi water supply have lesser fluoride levels but still more than 70% of people show the symptoms of dental fluorosis which can be attributed to irregular supply and inadequate utilization of Dharoi water as mentioned above.

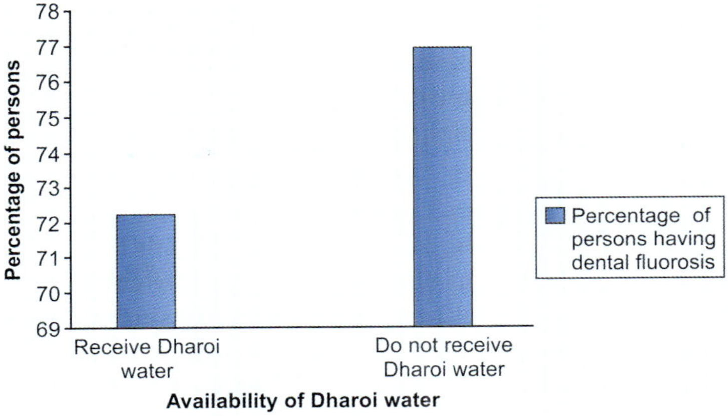

Figure 5.5: Prevalence of DF in relation to availabilty of Dharoi water

Table 5.13: Prevalence of DF in villages which do not receive supply of Dharoi water

Villages without Dharoi water supply	*Averave water fluoride in IWMI study*	*Average fluoride levels in 4 villages*	*Percentage of dental fluorosis*
Rajgarh	5.6	5.6	76.9%
Hansapur	4.10		
Ruppur	6.00		
Sojintra	6.50		

Table 5.14: Prevalence of DF in villages which receive supply of Dharoi water

Villages with Dharoi water supply	*Average water fluoride in IWMI study*	*Average fluoride levels in 6 villages*	*Percentage of dental fluorosis*
Mudana	1.28	2.8	72.2%
Pachakvada	0.99		
Surpura	1.01		
Karanpur	1.89		
Macchava	5.6		
Karsanpura	6.10		

Table 5.15: Grades of DF in relation to supply of Dharoi water

Supply of Dharoi water	*Total no. of persons examined*	*Persons having DF % (n)*	*Mild DF % (n)*	*Moderate DF % (n)*	*Severe DF % (n)*	*Absent % (n)*	*Not identified % (n)*
Receive Dharoi water	169(282)	72.2(240)	54.4(122)	15.4(92)	2.4(26)	16.6(4)	11.2(28)
Don't receive Dharoi water	113(282)	76.9(166)	29.2(87)	40.7(33)	7.1(46)	7.1 (8)	15.9(8)

Age Group Variation of Dental Fluorosis

It was observed that in almost all the age groups right from 8 years upto 62 years have almost 80% of the people showing the symptoms of dental fluorosis. The dental fluorosis in adults can be explained by the fact due to the entry of the fluoride when they were children or adolescent.

In the children and adolescent persons from the age group of 8 to 19 years also shows almost 80% of people showing dental fluorosis symptoms. This fact itself proves that people are still using fluoride rich water which can be further attributed to the irregular supply and inadequate utilization of Dharoi water as mentioned above.It can be further proven by the fact that the people are using blend of Dharoi and Borewell water for drinking and cooking purpose.

Table 5.16: Prevalence of DF in different age groups

Age group in years	*Total no. of persons examined*	*Total no. of persons having DF*	*Percentage of persons having DF*
<8	5	0	0
8–18	43	34	79.1
19–29	41	33	80.5
30–40	38	33	86.8
41–51	40	35	87.5
52–62	56	45	80.4
>62	59	29	49.2

Grades of Dental Fluorosis in different Age Groups

Mild Fluorosis is maximum in persons between 8 to 29 age groups which show that fluoride is still entering in their body. Moderate fluorosis is maximum in people between 52 to 62 age groups because the persons of this particular age group would have consumed more fluoride during their children and adolescent phase as shown in Tables 5.16 and 5.17.

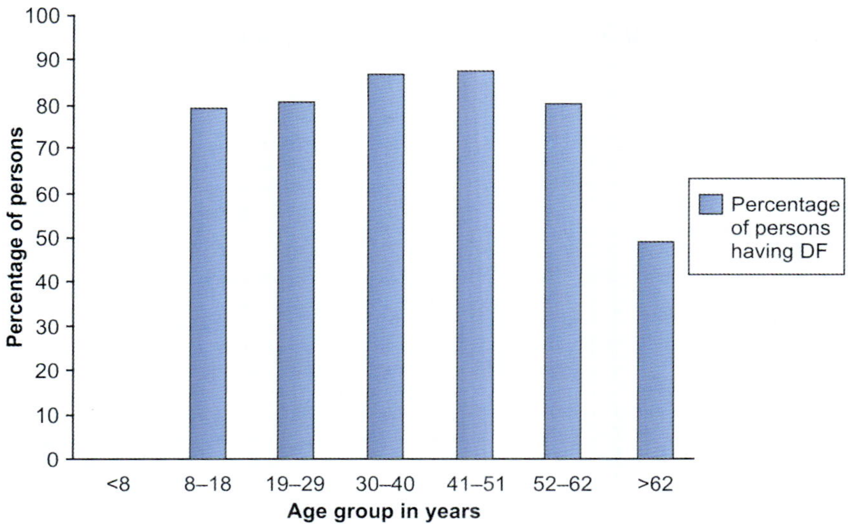

Figure 5.6: Prevalence of DF in different age groups

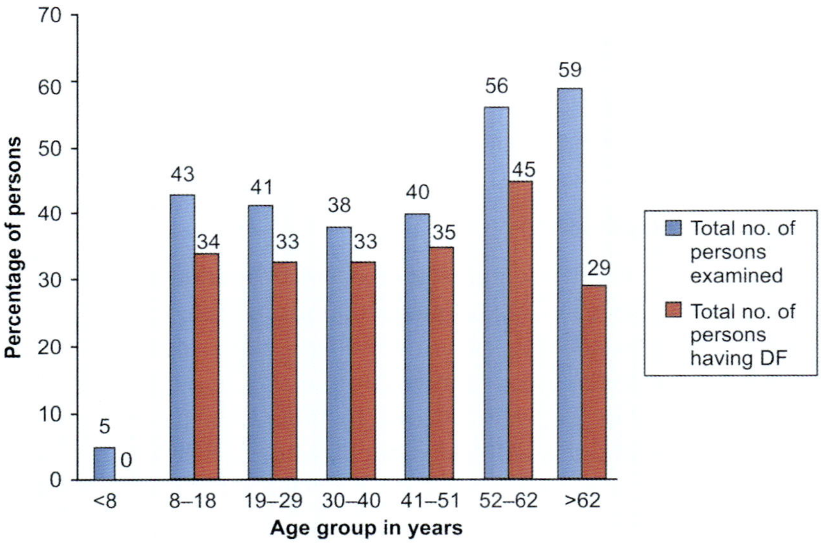

Figure 5.7: Variation of DF in different age group

Table 5.17: Grades of DF in different age groups

Age group in years	*Persons examined % (n)*	*Persons having DF % (n)*	*Mild DF % (n)*	*Moderate DF % (n)*	*Severe DF % (n)*	*Absent % (n)*	*NA %(n)*
<8	1.8 (5)	0 (0)	0 (0)	0 (0)	0 (0)	1.8 (5)	0 (0)
8–18	15.2 (43)	79.1 (34)	8.2 (23)	3.5 (10)	0.4 (1)	3.2 (9)	0 (0)
19–29	14.5 (41)	80.5 (33)	8.5 (24)	2.8 (8)	0.4 (1)	2.8 (8)	0 (0)
30–40	13.5 (38)	86.8 (33)	7.1 (20)	4.3 (12)	0.4 (1)	1.8(5)	0 (0)
41–51	14.2 (40)	87.5 (35)	6.7 (19)	5 (14)	0.7 (2)	0.4 (1)	1.4 (4)
52–62	20 (56)	80.4 (45)	6.7 (19)	7.4 (21)	1.8 (5)	1.8 (5)	2.1 (6)
>62	21 (59)	49.2 (29)	7.1 (20)	2.5 (7)	0.7 (2)	1.1 (3)	9.6 (27)

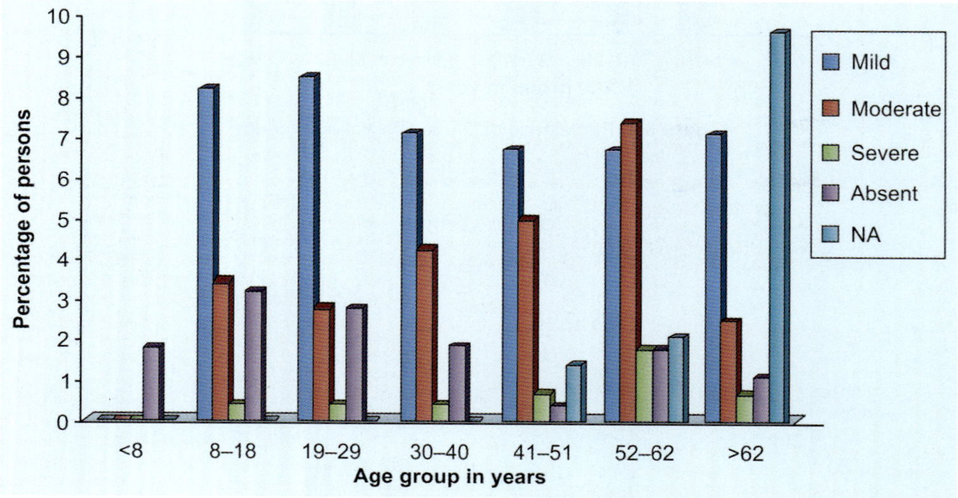

Figure 5.8: Grades of DF in different age groups

Musculoskeletal Fluorosis/Disorders

In 100 families out of 473 family members, there were 143 patients suffering from at least one of the five symptoms of fluorosis. It means that more than one person in a family is victim of fluorosis. The prevalence rate of musculoskeletal fluorosis was 30.2%. Out of this 19.6% or 28 person can't even walk properly. Around 58% of people can't bend forward easily and 67.8% can't sit up properly as shown in Table 5.19.They cannot move without some personal help or without hand-stick. Others, whose severity was found less could manage their daily chore with lot of pains, as complained by most of them. It's really a painful scenario in the villages!

Out of 143 patients only 53% or 76 persons took medical treatment; rest either could not afford or did not believe in medication to cure their pain.

Table 5.18: Symptomwise variation of MSD in afflicted persons

Symptoms of musculoskeletal fluorosis	*No. of persons*
Can't bend forward easily	83
Sit-ups not possible	97
Can't touch chin with chest	103
Can't touch back of head by hands	59
Unable to walk or move	28
Took medication	76

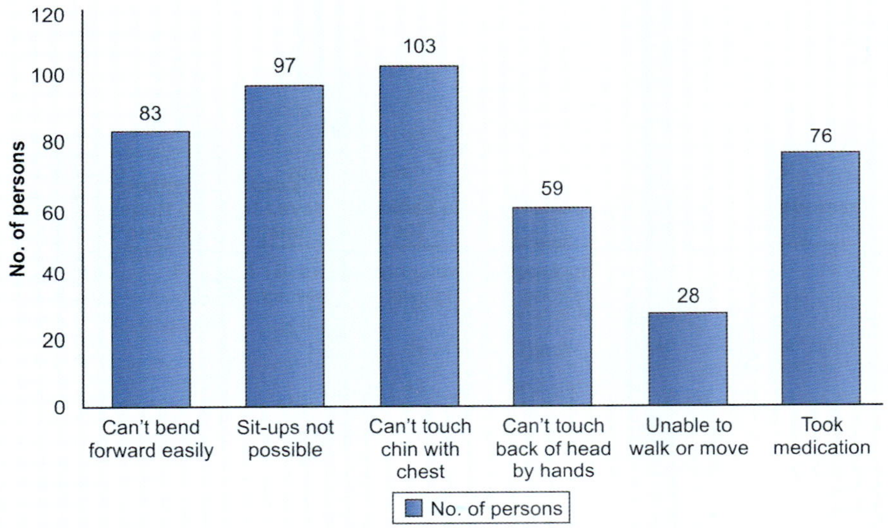

Figure 5.9: Symptomwise variation of MSD in a afflicted persons

Table 5.19: Variation of symptoms of MSD in afflicted persons

Symptoms of musculoskeletal fluorosis	*No. of persons*	*Percentage of symptoms*
Percent of afflicted persons of 473 family members	473	30.2
Total afflicted persons (143)	143	100.0
Can't bend forward easily	83	58.0
Sit-ups not possible	97	67.8
Can't touch chin with chest	103	72.0
Can't touch back of head by hands	59	41.3

Due to musculoskeletal fluorosis, the afflicted persons can't even do their normal activities as mentioned below. Majority of persons can't lift load and can't do cycling thus indirectly diminishing their working ability and earning capacity as shown in Table 5.20. In this survey, it was evident that there was average 60% decline in the earning capacity in the fluorosis afflicted people which is proven by the above mentioned facts.

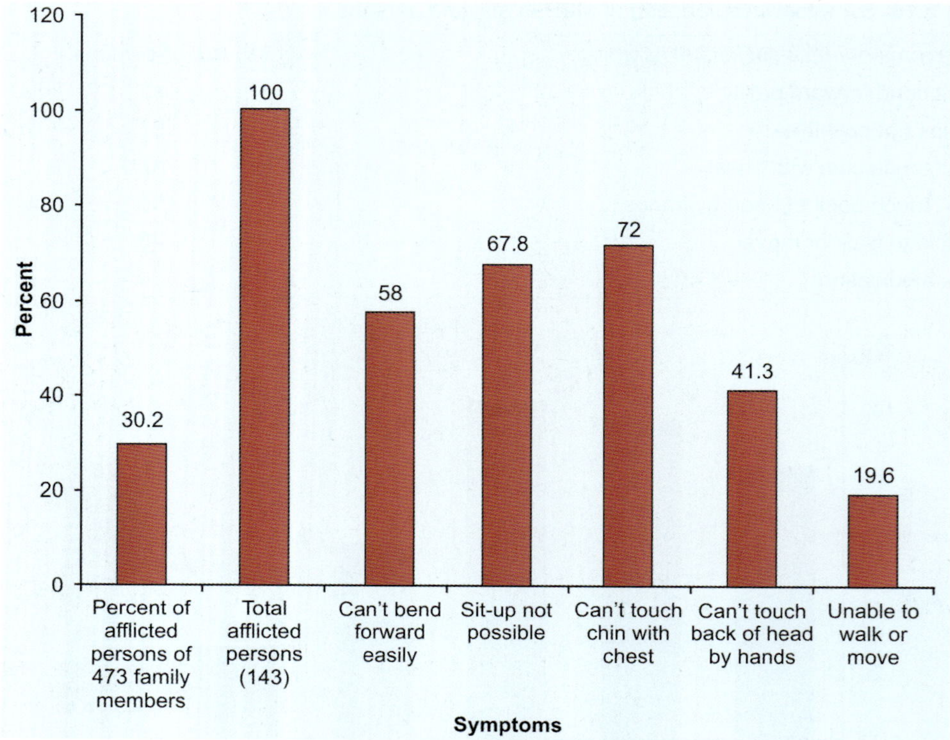

Figure 5.10: Variation of symptoms of MSD in afflicted persons

Table 5.20: Restriction of physical activities in afflicted persons

Various activities which can't be performed by patients	*No. of persons*
Can't do cycling	129
Can't walk in the field	65
Can't wipe floors	113
Can't lift load	132
Can't take care of cattle in home	110
Can't take care of children in home	32

Prevalence of Early Warning Signals of Fluorosis, i.e. Gastric Problems

This analysis of gastric problems was absent in **Shah and Indu.**

The hundred families were surveyed for gastric problems. It was observed that Out of 61 families receiving Dharoi water 41 families i.e. 67.2 % suffers from gastric problems as shown in Table 5.21. Out of 39 families which don't receive Dharoi water supply 18 families, i.e. 46.2% have gastric problems as shown in Table 5.22.

Table 5.21: Gastric problems in the afflicted families receiving Dharoi water

Total no. of families who receive Dharoi water = 61	*Families having gastric problems*				
	Diarrhea	*Pain in stomach*	*Constipation*	*Gas formation*	*Total no. and percentage of families having gastric trouble*
No. of families	2	13	12	14	41
Percentage of families	3.3	21.3	19.7	23.0	67.2

Table 5.22: Gastric problems in the afflicted families not receiving Dharoi water

Total no. of families who don't receive Dharoi water = 39	*Families having gastric problems*				
	Diarrhea	*Pain in stomach*	*Constipation*	*Gas formation*	*Total no. and percentage of families having gastric trouble*
No. of families	0	3	6	9	18
Percentage of families	0.0	7.7	15.4	23.1	46.2

It was also observed that out of 100 families questioned for gastric problems, 59 families had gastric problems and out of that 19 families said that it is due to water source like bore well or mixture of bore well and Dharoi water as shown in Table 5.23.

Table 5.23: Gastric problems in the families in relation to water source

Symptoms	*No. of families*	*Water source*
Diarrhea	2	1
Pain in stomach	16	5
Constipation	18	6
Gas problems	23	7

Majority of the families that is almost 70% complains of gas problems and constipation as shown in Figure 5.11 which are considered as early warning signals of fluorosis as quoted by **Dr A K Susheela**.

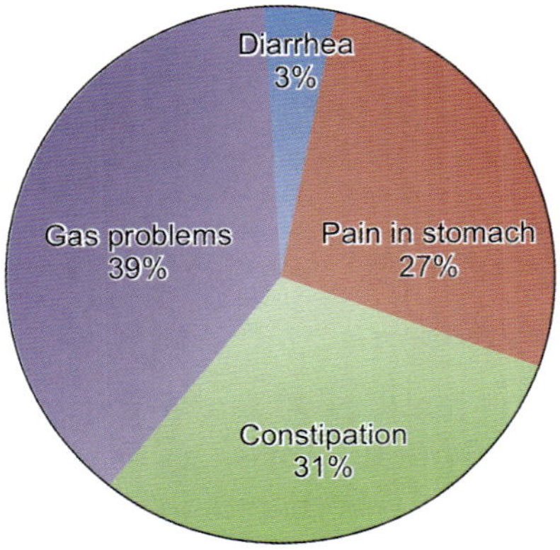

Figure 5.11: Gastric problems in afflicted families

Habits

It was observed that out of 100 families, 75 families are in the habit of taking tobacco, gutkha, supari, hajmola and Jaljeera. About 60% of the families are in the habit of Tobacco chewing as shown in Table 5.24.

Table 5.24: Study of families in terms of variation of different habits

Habits	Tobacco	Gutkha	Supari	Jaljeera	Hajmola
No.of families	45	18	4	0	8

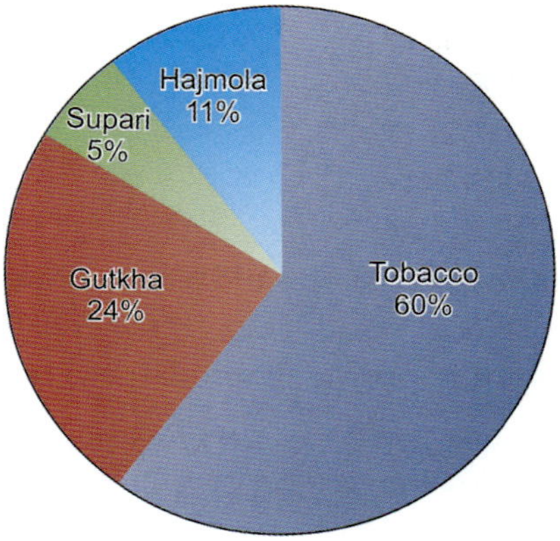

Figure 5.12: Study of families in terms of variation of habits

Awareness of Drinking Water

Opinion about Water Quality

In this survey the opinion of the respondents of the 100 families was taken regarding quality of the water used by them for drinking purposes. Around 67% of them said that the water they drink is of good quality and 32% of them said that it is of bad quality as shown in Table 5.25.

Table 5.25: Study of families in terms of perception about water quality

Perception of water quality	Good	Bad	None
No. of families	67	32	1

Awareness about RO water and Fluorosis

It was observed that out of 100 families 46 families have awareness about RO water and 8 families have awareness about fluorosis.Out of 46 families, 43 families drink RO water as shown in Table 5.26. It reveals that majority of the people still do not know about fluorosis.

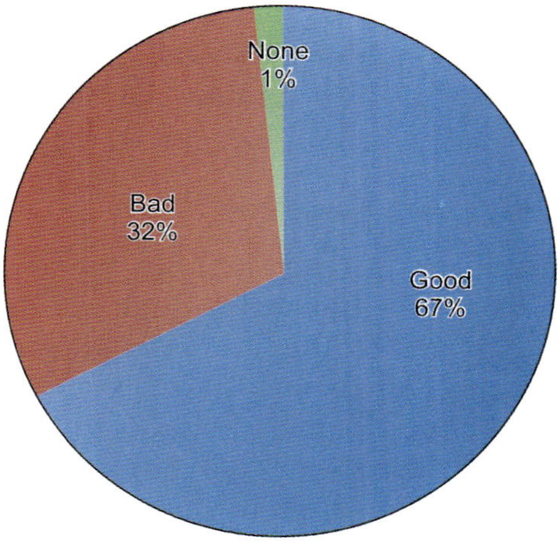

Figure 5.13: Study of families in terms of perception about water quality

Table 5.26: Study of families in terms of awareness about RO water and fluorosis

Awareness	RO water	Fluorosis
No. of families	46	8

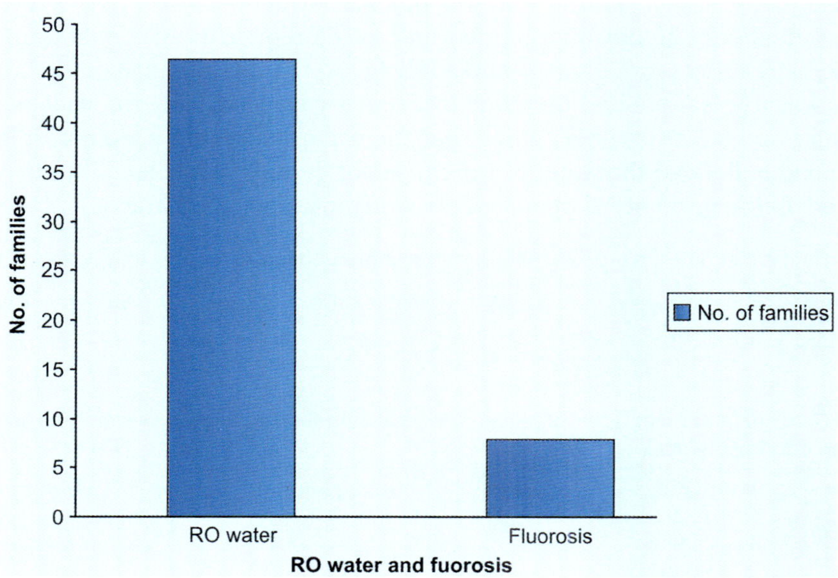

Figure 5.14: Study of families in items of awareness about RO water and fluorosis

Those families who use RO water were of the opinion that there was a difference in the quality of water between the water supplied in the village and the packaged drinking water. These families were using this water after they were advised either by doctor or friends or relatives. Some families even demanded subsidy on RO water. Around 20 families were willing to spend money for packaged RO water. Majority of the families couldn't afford to spend money on RO water. About 92% of the families had 'no-idea' about causes of fluorosis and 95% also did not know that anybody got cured or recovered from the sufferings of fluorosis after using demineralized water.

Perception of 'Good' water and 'Fluorosis'

In this survey, the feedback was also taken about the perception of respondents regarding fluorosis and its consequences through six different queries. Nearly 89% respondents had agreed that skeletal fluorosis severely reduced the capacity for work and earning income. About 80% had agreed that dental fluorosis is a major problem for young people, especially girls, because it reduces their self-confidence. Around 78% of the families agree that there is difficulty in marriages because of dental fluorosis. However, there was no such strong opinion that the skeletal fluorosis reduces the patient's interaction with other members of the community and leads to loneliness or isolation. Reason may be mostly people stay in a joint-family, or there are relatives and neighbors around the afflicted person. There is a community/family bond still prevailing in Indian village-life that may be working for not feeling so much lonely even though an afflicted person is not able to move much.

Further, there was no strong opinion or rather only 49% strongly agree with the perception that better quality of drinking water would reduce the skeletal fluorosis. At the same time, they agree (strongly 40% and softly (42%) that the damage in the body due to 'fluorosis' was irreversible and no medicinal remedy was available for skeletal fluorosis. Furthermore about 53% strongly agree that the water causes ugly teeth and joint pain. Hence, a solid belief that the water is 'the cause' for dental and skeletal fluorosis is still to be 'hatched' in the mind of the people of the study location in Gujarat.

Table 5.27: Study of families in terms of perception regarding the water causes ugly teeth and joint pain

Perception	Strongly agree	Agree	Do not know	Disagree	Strongly disagree
No. of families	53	19	14	14	0

Table 5.28: Study of families in terms of perception regarding skeletal fluorosis severely reduces capacity for work and earning income

Perception	Strongly agree	Agree	Do not know	Disagree	Strongly disagree
No. of families	4	89	6	1	0

Table 5.29: Study of families in terms of perception regarding better quality drinking water would reduce skeletal fluorosis

Perception	Strongly agree	Agree	Do not know	Disagree	Strongly disagree
No. of families	49	25	16	10	0

Table 5.30: Study of families in terms of perception regarding the damage in your body due to 'fluorosis,' which is irreversible and no medicinal remedy for skeletal fluorosis

Perception	Strongly agree	Agree	Do not know	Disagree	Strongly disagree
No.of families	40	42	15	3	0

Table 5.31: Study of families in terms of perception regarding difficulty in marriages because of dental fluorosis

Perception	Strongly agree	Agree	Do not know	Disagree	Strongly disagree
No. of families	9	78	6	7	0

Comparative Analysis with IWMI Study

According to IWMI study, out of total population of 28425, there were 4590 patients suffering from at least one of the five symptoms of fluorosis. It means that more than one person in a family is victim of fluorosis. The prevalence rate of musculoskeletal fluorosis was 16.1%. Among 4590 affected persons 14% or 643 cannot even walk properly and more than 64% per cent cannot situp and bend forward properly in Gujarat. They cannot move without some personal help or without hand-stick. Others, whose severity was found less could manage their daily chore with lot of pains, complained almost all of them. It is really a painful scenario in the villages! Only 4% of the total population and about 23% of the afflicted persons took medical treatment; rest 77% either could not afford or did not believe in medication to cure their pain.Out of these 28,425 people nearly 36% or 10,126 persons were also suffering from dental fluorosis (DF).

According to the present research study, the prevalence rate of musculoskeletal fluorosis is 30.2%. By taking into consideration, the fact in this study that only 473 persons of the 100 families have been checked for the symptoms of musculoskeletal fluorosis as compared to 28425 persons in IWMI study, it can be concluded that the prevalence rate of musculoskeletal fluorosis (30.2% in present study and 16.1% in IWMI study) is still higher and there is negligible effect of Dharoi water supply or other preventive measures in curbing the fluorosis in these villages of North Gujarat. Similarly the prevalence of dental fluorosis in this study is 74.1% amongst 282 people examined as compared to IWMI study where the prevalence was 30.2% amongst 28425 persons examined. In IWMI study the Dean's Index criteria was not used and the various cases of mild fluorosis were not taken into account. This can be further explained by the fact that the person having non-discolored tooth can also be diagnosed as mild dental fluorotic case according to Dean's index criteria. In this study, the mild fluorosis was present in maximum number of persons that is almost 44.3%, which is quite significant. "Dean advised that when the average child in a community has mild fluorosis, . . . it begins to constitute a public health problem warranting increasing consideration" (Dean 1942, p. 29)." NRC 2006 p 106.

Thus, it can be concluded that the fluorosis is still a major public health problem in these villages of North Gujarat.

Table 5.32: Comparison of musculoskeletal fluorosis in IWMI study and present study

	IWMI study	*Present study*
Total no. of people examined (%)	28425 (100)	473 (100)
Any one symptom of Va/fluorosis/MSD present (afflicted) (%)	4590 (16.1)	143 (30.2)
Can not touch chest with chin (%)	992 (3.5)	103 (21.8)
Cannot bend forward easily (%)	2956 (10.4)	83 (17.5)
Can not do sit ups (%)	2979 (10.5)	97 (20.5)
Cannot touch back of the head with hand (%)	1515 (5.3)	59 (12.5)
Crippled/unable to walk (%)	643 (2.3)	28 (5.9)
Taking medical treatment (%)	1046 (3.7)	76 (16)

Table 5.33: Comparison of dental fluorosis in IWMI study and present study

	Total no. of people examined (%)	*Dental fluorosis (%)*
IWMI study	28425 (100)	10126 (35.6)
Present study	282 (100)	209 (74.1)

Note

In this survey, the views of the Doctors and Dentists practising in these endemic areas of North Gujarat were also captured. The fourteen doctors were surveyed regarding various aspects about fluorosis. Out of 14 doctors, majority of Doctors that is nine doctors said that the number of reporting cases of fluorosis have decreased since last 3 to 4 years after supply of Dharoi water. Majority of the doctors that is nine doctors were of the view that the joint or back pain in the people of these villages is because of fluoride in water. Majority of them suggested the use of demineralised water as a mitigation measure to curb fluorosis. Some of the doctors also stress the use of iron and calcium to mitigate effects of the fluorosis.

The role of nutrition for prevention and mitigation of fluorosis is highly important as reported in our field study by Dr DJ Bhavsar (MBBS, MS) who has been practicing in Unjha since last few decades on fluorosis has several evidences of patients recovering from some symptoms of musculoskeletal fluorosis due to interaction of enhanced nutrition. With regard to fluorosis the main nutrition requirements can be summarized as those of calcium, magnesium and vit. C as cited by **Dr Susheela, A K and Raja Reddy.**

Hence by all these observations it can be said that fluorosis is mainly related to water. But it has relations with nutrients and dietary factor also.

Conclusion

This study concludes that there is still very grim condition of fluorosis in these ten villages of North Gujarat. The dental fluorosis is very much prevalent in these areas. There seems to be insignificant improvement in the fluorosis condition in these families. The mitigation measure taken to curb fluorosis like water supply from Dharoi dam seems to be inefficient due to irregular and dirty supply of the water supplemented by the non-usage of Dharoi water by the people due to misconceptions attached to it as mentioned above. There seems to be other factors also involved rather than water alone, in causing fluorosis. Diet can be a major such factor.

One of the MDG that is MDG number seven (ensure environmental sustainability) in context to India is "the proportion of population without sustainable access to safe drinking water and sanitation is to be halved by 2015" but it seems to be a distant dream especially in these villages of North Gujarat. The fluorosis doesn't cause mortality but it makes the person crippled socially as well as physically which is more deplorable rather than being dead. The fluorosis should be taken seriously as the national agenda by the government as it is incurable but it can be prevented by providing safe drinking water supplemented with good nutrition. We should never forget that fluorosis is related to water and safe drinking water is one of the basic needs of human being. Fluorosis is also related to nutrition so diet rich in calcium, protein, vitamin C, etc. can alleviate the detrimental consequences of fluorosis. Hence safe and quality drinking water along with good nutrition can help in curbing fluorosis in these villages.

Fluorosis, which was considered to be a problem related to teeth only, has now turned up to be a serious health hazard. It seriously affects bones and problems like joint pain, muscular pains, etc. are its wellknown manifestations. It not only affects the body of a person but also renders them socially and culturally crippled. In spite of the progressive spread of disease so far no established data exists to determine the extent of disease, no specialized water testing facilities are available and even the doctors do not have specific orientation to corelate the disease with specific symptoms. In these areas the response of the people is reactive rather then pro-active.

The present study acts as a pointer to public health physicians, dentists, chemists, planners, administrators, engineers and water supply authorities. The information furnished can be utilized as preliminary data, and a well-designed epidemiological investigation can be undertaken at taluk level and district level to confirm and assess dental fluorosis and to evaluate the risk factors associated with the condition in the study region.

"I sincerely hope that, besides the general public, policy makers and health officials, in the interest of the nation and the people they are sworn to serve, will learn from reading this book to recognize and desist from the 'madness' being exercised by 'fluoridation of drinking water.' "In the meantime, many people using fluoridated drinking water will have illness with fatigue that is not relieved by sleep. Hopefully, this book will help those so affected to realize that their health is in their own hands and that a cure is possible. Feedback from readers will be welcomed by the author.

Limitations

In this study, Recall bias may be there as certain questions were asked about perception of relief in pain after supply of Dharoi water. Dental fluorosis develops in an individual during the time of teeth calcification and the fluoride content of water during that period is of prime importance. There are also shortcomings of Dean's Index of Fluorosis, principally its inability to measure fluorosis in different tooth surfaces. As it has been traditionally used, it also does not permit specifying the cosmetic importance of the most severe fluorosis detected in a dentition. This population based survey only represents small fraction of population. A larger scale study would have been more appropriate. Finally water samples from each village were not collected and screened due to lack of resources and the fluoride data of water and the subjects chosen for the study from each of these villages were taken from the **IWMI's Study** in 2004 under the name of **"Fluorosis in Gujarat: A Disaster Ahead".**

Recommendations

The high fluoride content in water is the main reason for the fluorosis in these villages. Hence, it requires synergistic action from health planners, health administrators, engineers and water supply authorities to supply safe drinking water with permissible limit of fluoride. The people of these villages are mostly using bore well water for drinking, which adds to the existing problem as it depletes the groundwater leading to excavate further deep for the bore well water. It is known that the content of fluoride in groundwater is directly proportional with the depth of water table. Hence, use of groundwater for drinking should be discouraged and be replaced by surface water.

Water supply from Dharoi dam being a safer source of surface water with permissible limits of fluoride was introduced in these villages as one of the mitigation measure to curb fluorosis. In hundred families studied, around 60% of families receive Dharoi water and 40% of families still don't receive Dharoi. Incidentally, those who are receiving still don't have regular supply. There are also other problems for irregular supply like pipeline leakage or lack of pressure or hefty bill payments to get Dharoi water. There were certain misconceptions linked to the non-utilization of Dharoi water like water is very cold and filthy and dirty. Some families said that it causes cough and has foul odor and taste. All these factors potentiate the inadequate utilization of Dharoi water. There is also the habit of mixing Dharoi water with bore well water in order to meet the daily demands of these families which should be discouraged.

Hence all these problems regarding irregular and dirty supply of Dharoi water should be sorted out urgently. The efforts should be made to provide safe and qualitative and regular supply of Dharoi water. The fluorosis may be related to the other factors like diet, etc. as mentioned in studies and papers like Fluoride and Fluorosis and Reversal of

Fluorosis in Children, etc. The further research is needed in this regard to understand the role of diet and nutrition in the prevention and treatment of fluorosis.

Overall, Recommendations of this study can be summarized as:

1. There should be adequate and regular supply of Dharoi water so that the community need not to mix Dharoi water with bore well water and thus they can rely on safe water for drinking purpose.
2. The proper attention should be paid to make Dharoi water potable for drinking (like water should be odorless, colorless, usable for domestic purposes and free from harmful chemical substances and pathogenic substances) so that the acceptability to the community is enhanced.
3. The awareness about fluorosis should be encouraged with involvement of community leaders to rectify the misconceptions regarding usage of Dharoi water.
4. The authentic efforts should be made to repair the broken pipelines supplying Dharoi water and other supply issues should also be sorted out.
5. The efforts should also be made to sort out administrative issues regarding supply of Dharoi water like hefty bill payments and regular supply.
6. The low cost, replicable technologies should be developed and experimented to make sure every one gets access to safe drinking water. It should also be our priority to demonstrate that fluorosis can be prevented if not cured and impress upon the government to make it a national policy to ensure safe drinking water as a fundamental right for every one.
7. The further research throwing light about sources of fluoride entry into the body like diet/ food items apart from water is desirable to comprehend the problem of fluorosis.
8. The further research is also needed to understand the role of nutrition in fluorosis and its effects or symptoms in body as it has been seen that in some areas having high fluoride levels don't suffer much clinically from fluorosis.

Fast Facts

- Fluoride ingestion is hazardous to health
- Besides drinking water, fluoride can enter the body through food, dental products, drugs and industrial emission
- Health complaints emanating from fluoride poisoning are of diverse nature
- Affliction of children due to fluoride poisoning are significantly different from adults
- In children the adverse effects commence from intra-uterine life, if the mother is exposed to high fluoride
- Infants with respiratory distress should be tested for fluoride in urine of the infant/ drinking water, blood and urine of the mother
- Fluoride ingestion by the infant from early developmental stages can lead to rickets, which may not respond to calcium and vitamin D treatment; unless the fluoride levels in urine/blood are lowered to normal range

- Fluorosis ranges in severity from mild to severe
- Permanent teeth are more susceptible to fluorosis than primary dentition
- The most susceptible age for fluorosis is between 15 and 30 months
- In children the discoloration seen on the permanent teeth may not necessarily be due to dental caries or dirty teeth
- The discoloration of the permanent teeth can be due to dental fluorosis
- Dental Fluorosis can be distinguished from dental caries and dirty teeth by the following yardsticks:

  In dental fluorosis, the discoloration is always horizontally aligned on the enamel surface; discoloration shall be away from the gums; the discoloration shall occur in teeth in pair (bilaterally symmetrical)
- Fluoride poisoning effects in adults can be tracked to soft tissue manifestations besides skeletal derangements
- Identifying fluorosis at early stages could potentially save millions of life if intial observations can be confirmed through fluoride test in blood and urine
- The importance of the confirmatory test is to catch the patients at the turning points, before the disease affects multiple organs and systems including bony rigidity and paralysis
- The prevailing social customs make most men in the fluorosis villages to remain at the same place right from birth using locally available high-fluoride water for both drinking and cooking. They develop progressively severe symptoms of fluorosis till death
- The prevailing social customs on the other hand make women to move from father's house to husband's house and in the process may move from a fluorosis area to a non-fluorosis area and vice versa
- Apart from this, women lose some additional fluoride through menstruation, offspring and lactation
- Between men and women, severity of skeletal fluorosis is therefore generally less in women than in men.

ANNEXURES

1. FLUOROSIS PHOTOGRAPHS

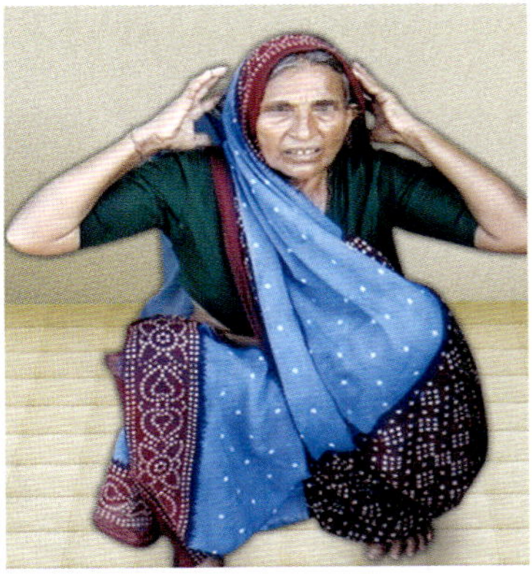

Musculoskeletal fluorosis
Champaben Chamar, 60F
Village Pachakvada

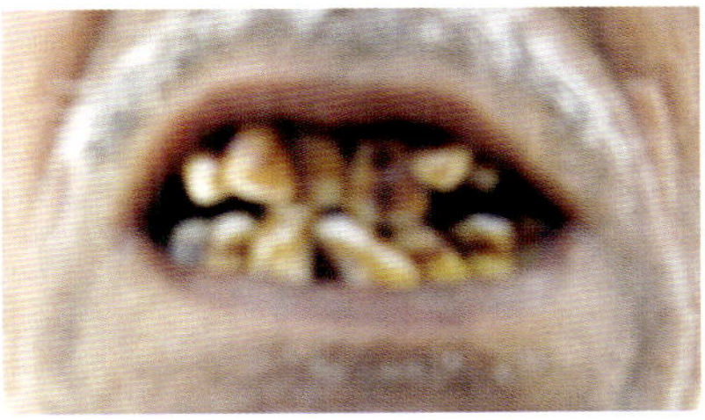

Dental fluorosis
Ishvarbhai Rabari
Village Sojintra

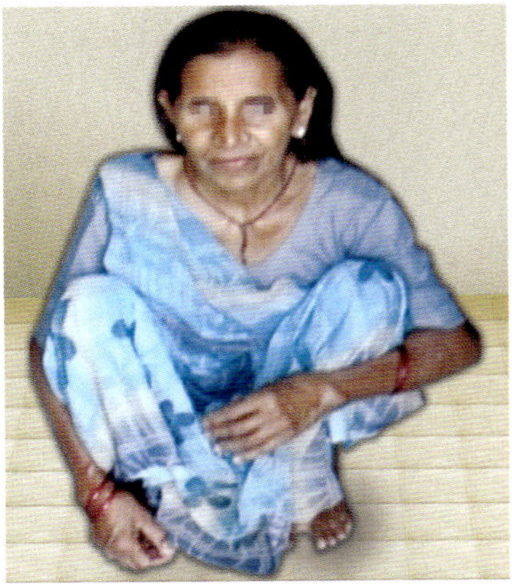

Crippled musculoskeletal fluorosis
Manguben Amrulal Patel
Village Surpura

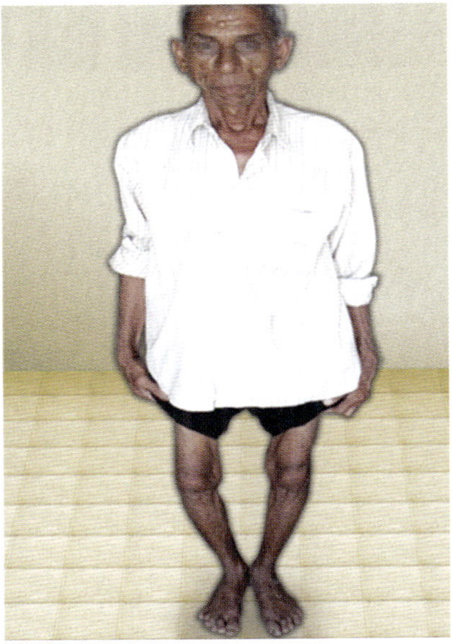

Musculoskeletal fluorosis
Manilal Lildas Patel
Village Karanpur

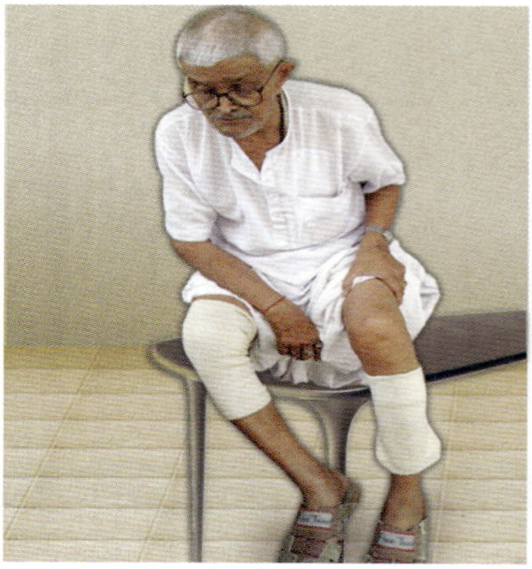

Musculoskeletal fluorosis
Manjibhai Patel
Village Ruppur

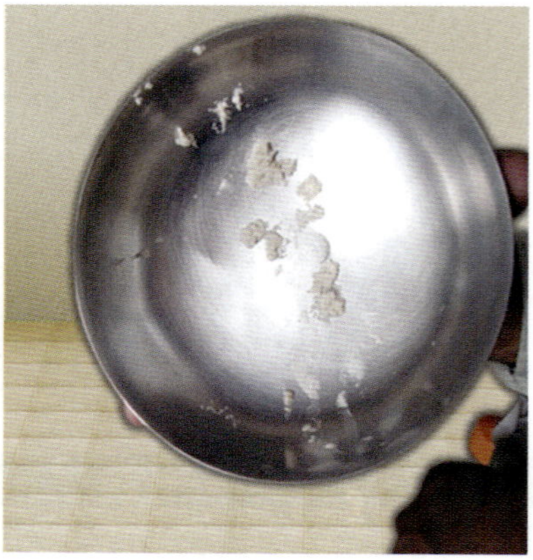

Salted tubewell water
Village Rajgarh

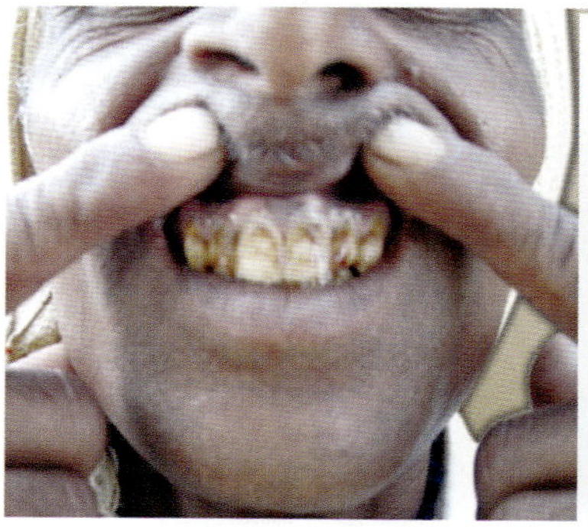

Dental fluorosis
Sataji Gemarji, Village Aadhava

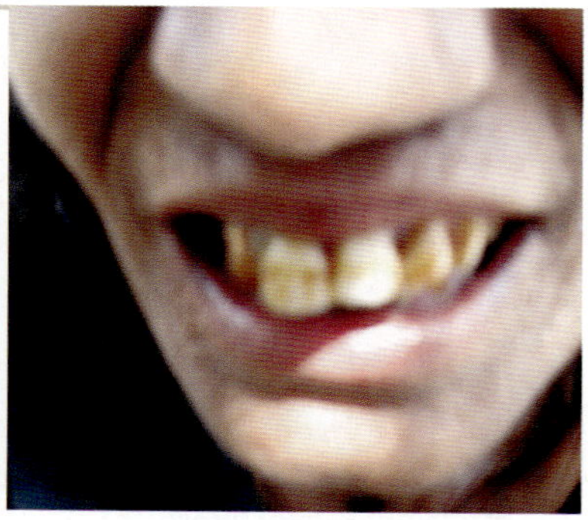

Dental fluorosis
Latjiben, Village Sojintra

2. FLUORIDE CONTENT IN AGRICULTURAL PRODUCTS AND OTHER EDIBLE ITEMS (FLUORIDE IN PPM)

Food item	*Place of study*	
	A. Kolkata [Sengupta and Pal (1971)]	*B. Mumbai [Lakdawala and Puneker (1973)]*
Fluoride content in drinking water (ppm)	0.4	0.15–0.48
Cereals and Tubers		
Cereal	4.6	2.59–3.3
Wheat	5.9	3.27–14.03
Rice	--	1.72–2.23
Maize	5.6	--
Pulses and Legumes		
Bengal gram	6.2	3.84–4.84
Green gram dal	2.5	2.34–4.84
Red gram dal	3.7	2.34–4.84
Soyabean	4.0	--
Leafy Vegetables		
Spinach	2.0	0.77–4.14
Cabbage	3.3	1.28–2.29
Amaranth leaves	5.8	4.91–7.14
Lettuce	5.7	--
Mint	4.8	--
Bathua leaves	6.3	--
Chowli leaves	--	1.79–7.33
Other Vegetables		
Cucumber	4.1	2.57–3.58
French beans	--	1.07–1.96
Tomato	3.4	1.00–2.08
Brinjal	1.2	1.62–2.48
Ladies finger	4.0	2.2–3.62
Snake gourd	2.3	2.16–3.44
Roots and Tubers		
Beet root	4.2	--
Carrot	4.1	1.9–4.9
Potato	2.8	1.27–2.92
Onion	3.7	1.00–3.00
Sweet potato	3.2	--

Food item	*Place of study*	
	A. Kolkata [Sengupta and Pal (1971)]	*B. Mumbai [Lakdawala and Puneker (1973)]*
Fruits		
Banana	2.9	0.84–1.58
Dates	4.5	--
Grapes	—	0.84–1.74
Figs	4.2	--
Mango	3.7	0.8–1.80
Apple	5.7	1.05–2.2
Guava	5.1	0.24–0.52
Nuts and Oil seeds		
Almond	4.0	—
Cashewnut	4.1	—
Coconut	4.4	—
Mustard seeds	5.7	—
Groundnut	5.1	—
Beverages		
Tea (dry leaves)	—	39.8–68.59
Tea infusion (1 gram boiled for 5 minutes in 125 mL water)	—	18.13–56.19
Tea infusion (1 gram in 125 mL) of hot water)	—	11.13–37.34
Aerated drinks	—	0.77–1.44
Coconut water	—	0.43–0.60
Spices and Condiments		
Corriander	2.3	—
Cumin seeds	1.8	—
Garlic	5.0	—
Ginger	2.0	—
Tamarind pulp	3.8	—
Termeric	3.3	—
Food from Animal sources		
Mutton	—	3.0–3.5
Beef	—	4.0–5.0
Pork	—	3.0–4.5
Fish	—	1.0–6.5

3. DEAN'S INDEX CRITERIA FOR DENTAL FLUOROSIS

Criteria for Dean's Fluorosis Index	
Score	**Criteria**
Normal	The enamel represents the usual translucent semivitriform type of structure. The surface is smooth, glossy and usually of a pale creamy white color.
Questionable	The enamel discloses slight aberrations from the translucency of normal enamel, ranging from a few white flecks to occasional white spots. This classification is utilized in those instances where a definite diagnosis of the mildest form of fluorosis is not warranted and a classification of "normal" is not justified.
Very mild	Small opaque, paper white areas scattered irregularly over the tooth but not involving as much as 25% of the tooth surface. Frequently included in this classification are teeth showing no more than about 1–2 mm of white opacity at the tip of the summit of the cusps of the bicuspids or second molars.
Mild	The white opaque areas in the enamel of the teeth are more extensive but do not involve as much as 50% of the tooth.
Moderate	All enamel surfaces of the teeth are affected, and the surfaces subject to attrition show wear. Brown stain is frequently a disfiguring feature.
Severe	Includes teeth formerly classified as "moderately severe and severe." All enamel surfaces are affected and hypoplasia is so marked that the general form of the tooth may be affected. The major diagnostic sign of this classification is discrete or confluent pitting. Brown stains are widespread and teeth often present a corroded-like appearance.

4. CALCIUM RICH FOOD (MG/100 G)

Ajwayan	1525	Imi	170	Rice bran	67
Til	1450	Bakri ka doodh	170	Bhindi	66
Skimmed milk powder	1370	Karonda	160	Sem	60
Mar (agathi)	1130	Mirch dry	160	Arwi ki dandi	60
Jira	1080	Methi	160	Bara sem	60
Khoa (skimmed buf milk)	990	Sarson-ka-sag	155	Murgi ka anda	60
Whole milk powder	950	Urad dal	154	Bhuna chana	58
Kantewali chaulai	800	Bakri ka gosht	150	Arhar, tender	57
Long dry	740	Haldi	150	Chane-ki-dal	56
Shalgam ka sag	710	Bathua sag	150	Sayan ki phalli	51
Hing	690	Dahi	149	Muli	50
Dhania	630	Pista	140	Zimikand	50
Phool gobee sag	626	Elaychi	130	Sem	50
Bachuva	520	Munakka	130	Fras bean	50

Rai	490	Guar ki phalli	130	Kathal seeds	50
Panner	480	Falsa	129	Lasson	50
Kali mirch	460	Mung	124	Supari	50
Coconut dry	400	Gay ka doodh	120	Kaju	50
Chaulai sag	397	Khajur	120	Amla	50
Chukandar ka sag	380	Kalni sag	110	Atta	48
Methi sag	395	Imli patte	101	Tamator	48
Kaddu ka sag	392	Sarson ki dandi	100	Pyaz (onion) big	46
Ari	380	Akhrot	100	Shakarkand, Sweet Potato	46
Chumli sag (arai keerai)	364	Katchua ka anda	93	Chotee gobee	43
Bargad ka phal	364	Chilgoza	91	Bajra	42
Madua (ragi)	344	Moong phali	90	Gehun	41
Chana sag	340	Neembu	90	Wheat gram	40
Gajar sag	340	Kishmish	87	Arwi	40
Samp machli	330	Bel (bael fruit)	85	Pyaz small	40
Kala til	300	Matar roasted	81	Mausambi	40
Lobia	290	Gadhe ka doodh	80	Rusbhary	40
Kulthi (horse gram)	287	Gud (cane)	80	Band gobee	39
Chironji	279	Lauki ka sag	80	Wheat bulgar (parboiled)	37
Mooli ka sag	265	Gajar	80	Amra	36
Rajmah	260	Anjeer	80	Phul gobi	33
Cholai-ki-dandi	260	Matar dry	79	Kharbooja	32
Bhatmas (soyabean)	240	Mung dal	75	Kangni(italian millet)	31
Pan ka patta	230	Lobia	77	Shalgam	30
Badam	230	Arhar dal	73	Mirch green	30
Bhains ka doodh	210	Palak	73	Lehson dry	30
Chana	202	Nimbu bada	70	Malta	30
Moth	202	Shahtoot	70	Suar ka gosht	30
Gendhri	200	Bathak ka anda	70	Lassi	30
Pudina	200	Masur dal	69	Makhan	00
Hara dhania	184	Gai ka ghosht	68		

5. VITAMIN C RICH FOOD (MG/100 G)

Amla	600	Bhindi	13
Shalgam ka sag	180	Lehson dry	13
Hara dhania	169	Bachuva	13
Mar (agathi)	135	Bara sem	12
Band gobee	124	Shahtoot	12
Mirch green	111	Ari	11
Chaulai sag	99	Lasson	11
Mooli ka sag	81	Pyaz (onion) big	11
Gajar sag	79	Cholai-ki-dandi	10
Chotee gobee	72	Gadhe ka doodh	10
Chukandar ka sag	70	Bel (bael fruit)	8
Neembu	63	Coconut dry	7
Phul gobi	56	Lobia	4
Malta	54	Pan ka patta	5
Methi sag	52	Anjeer	5
Mirch dry	50	Skimmed milk powder	5
Mausambi	50	Whole milk powder	4
Guar ki phalli	49	Chana	3
Shalgam	43	Imli patte	3
Nimbu bada	39	Gajar	3
Kalni sag	37	Arwi ki dandi	3
Bathua sag	35	Jira	3
Kantewali chaulai	33	Imli	3
Sarson-ka-sag	33	Khajur	3
Rusbhary	30	Samp machli	3
Palak	28	Moth	2
Tamator	27	Pyaz small	2
Pudina	27	Suar ka gosht	2
Sem	27	Gay ka doodh	2
Kharbooja	26	Chane-ki-dal	
Arhar, tender	25	Kulthi (horse gram)	
Shakarkand,sweet potato	24	Munakka	
Fras bean	24	Kishmish	
Falsa	22	Bhains ka doodh	
Amra	21	Bakri ka doodh	
Muli	17	Dahi	
Kathal seeds	14		

6. VILLAGE QUESTIONNAIRE

India Natural Resource Economic and Management Foundation (INREM), Anand
Tel: 02692-262385 and
Indian Institute of Public Health (IIPH), Gandhinagar. Tel: 079-40240444

Respondent's Identification (Sarpanch, Talati or Any Knowledgeable Person of the Village)

Name of the Respondent:	
Sarpanch/Talati/any knowledgeable person of the village:	
Address:	
Pin Code:	
Tele: (STD Code:) No.:	Mobile No:

1. Total population of village: ....; Total area of village .... Ha
2. Does the village have a water supply system? Yes/No
3. Does the village get water from Dharoi water supply system? Yes/No
4. If Yes above, from when did Dharoi water start supply to village? Year ....
5. Does the village panchayat have groundwater for water source? Yes/No
6. Are there separate pipes for supplying Dharoi water and groundwater to village? Yes/No
7. If Yes above, is this true for entire village? Yes/No
8. Is Dharoi water mixed with groundwater? Yes/No
9. If Yes above, in what proportion is this mixing done? .... % of Dharoi water
10. What is the frequency of Dharoi water supply?

Season	***Frequency (once in how many days)***
Monsoon	
Winter	
Summer	

11. What is the fluoride concentration of groundwater in the village? .... mg/L
12. What is the TDS concentration of groundwater in the village? ....

7. FAMILY QUESTIONNAIRE

Family Code			
D	T	V	Form No

Qs – 1. Queries from Selected Families

Respondent's Identification:

District:	Taluka:	Village:
Name of the Respondent:		Caste:
Address:		
		Pin Code:
Telephone: (LL) STD Code:	No.	Mob.:
Relation with Head of the Family:	Sex:	Age:

1. Family Particulars

1.1	Age	<6	6–12	12–18	18–40	40–60	> 60	Total (Male) Members
	Age	<6	6–12	12–18	18–40	40–60	> 60	Total (Female) Members

1.2	Income Sources in the Family: Please ✓ tick	Farming	Service/ Teacher	Business	Others

1.3	*Education among family members: Write number of members:*						
	NA <5 years	Not at all	Non-SSC	SSS-HSC	Graduate	Postgraduate	Others

2. Water Supply in the Family

2.1 What is the source of water for your family?

Supply Source	***Distance***	***Main use for D, B, W and C****	***Do you store daily? Y/N***	***Remarks***
Tubewell: Panchayat				
Tubewell: Private/Agri				
Others/RO/Hand pump/Open well				

* D = Drinking, B = Bathing, W = Washing and C = Cattle

2.2 Do you receive Dharoi water? ... Yes/No

2.3 If Yes, since when?

2.4 How frequently do you receive Dharoi water? (Once in .... Days)

2.5 Do you think Dharoi water is of good quality? Yes/No

2.6 When you do not receive Dharoi water, what other source of water do you use? Tanker/Borewell/Package water/others............

2.7 What is the proportion of Dharoi water in your drinking and cooking purpose in a year?

a. 0–25%, b. 25–50%, c. 50–75%, d. 75%+

2.8 Since getting Dharoi water, do you observe changes in any health symptoms in your family?

Sl. No.	*Symptoms*	*Remained same*	*Decreased*	*Increased*	*Remarks, if any*
1					
2					
3					
4					

2.9 Do you see changes in dental problems of children since Dharoi water has come? Yes/No

3. Clinical Examination of Dental Fluorosis (DF) (Here a thorough examination of family members will be done to diagnose DF)

	Sl. No.					
	1	*2*	*3*	*4*	*5*	*6*
Name						
Relation						
Sex						
Age						
Education						
Discoloration of teeth towards apical, middle, and cervical parts						
Any coloring of teeth Yes/No						
Any bleeding from gums Yes/No						
Severity — absent, mild, moderate, severe						
Any treatment done for DF						

4. Questions Related to Musculoskeletal Fluorosis

4.1. Is there anyone suffering from 'Va' or MSD or Fluorosis? Yes/No, If yes ...

	Sl. No.		
	1	*2*	*3*
Name			
Relation			
Sex			
Age			
Education			
Vocation			
Since when? Year			
Bending forward easily Y/N			
Sit-Ups possible Y/N			
Touching chin with chest Y/N			
Touching back of head by hands Y/N			
Unable to walk or move Y/N			
Medication Yes/No			
Expenses on scraping teeth in case of DF last year (Rs)			
Expenses on MSD in case in last year (Rs)			

4.2. How was the diagnosis done for 'Va' or MSD of the above person/s?

a. By a doctor: Yes/No
b. By others: Yes/No
c. X-ray done: Yes/No
d. Urine examination done: Yes/No
e. Any other examination done to detect fluorosis? If 'Yes' give details:
f. Was any other examination done to diagnose fluorosis? If 'Yes' give details:
g. Did your doctor say that the 'Va' is due to the quality of water? Yes/No
h. If 'yes' did he mention about 'fluoride' in the water you drink? Yes/No

4.3. Ask the 'Va'/MSD/Fluorosis afflicted person/s mentioned in Q. 4.1 above about his/her inability to do the following:

		Sl. No. as in Q 4.1		
		1	*2*	*3*
	Name			
	(a) Relation with respondent			
	(b) Sex			
	(c) Age			

Contd...

Contd...

Write—Yes/No	Do Cycling			
	Walk in the field			
	Wipe floors			
	Lift load			
	Take care of cattle in home			
	Take care of children in home			
	Do some other work (specify)			

4.4. Working Capacity: Can you do your normal duties or work? Yes/No
- If 'No' write the following

	Sl. No. as in Q 4.1		
	1	**2**	**3**
Name			
Relation			
Sex			
Earning capacity declined by percentage			
What was your occupation? Farming/Agri. Lab./ Service			
Since how long you are not able to work: year/month			
What was your last earning per day/per month? Rs.			
What is your present earning, per day/per month/per year? Rs.			

5. Do you have any other complaints other than above Q. 3 and Q, 4 in your family?

If yes then write below:

	Is due to water? Yes/No	***If Yes, which source?***	***How frequent in a year?***	***What remedy you take?***
Diarrhea: Yes/No				
Pain in stomach: Yes/No				
Constipation: Yes/No				
Gas formation: Yes/No				

6. Diet and Nutrition

6.1. Diet: Veg or Non-veg = V/NV

6.2. What is frequency of intake of food? in hours ...

6.3. Current food practices:

Breakfast (morning)	***Lunch***	***Anything like snacks***	***Dinner***

6.4. What food grains/vegetables do you eat?

Sl. No.	Whether grown locally? Yes/No
Wheat	
Bajri	
Rice	
Vegetable	

6.5. Do you or anyone in your family take?—tobacco, gutkha, supari, jaljeera, hajmola

6.6. Which toothpaste you use? Please give name =

7. Awareness of Drinking Good Water

1	What is your opinion about the water you drink?	Good	Bad	None
2	Are you aware of RO Water?	Yes	No	
3	If 'Yes' do you drink RO Water?	Yes	No	
4	If 'Yes' do you find any difference between RO water and non-RO water?	Yes	No	
5	If 'Yes' how much would you like to spend for RO water for your family? Rs. per month:	Rs.		
6	If you do not get RO water, do you purify drinking water by any other means: If so, give details:			
7	Have heard of "Fluorosis? If 'yes' do you have any idea of what causes 'Fluorosis'? Details -			
8	It is said that presence of fluoride in water causes fluorosis. Do you know anybody who was suffering from fluorosis, but recovered after using good /RO water?	Yes	No	

8. Perception Survey of the Respondent

		Strongly agree	Agree	Do not know	Disagree	Strongly disagree
1	The water we drink causes ugly teeth and joint pain.					
2	Dental fluorosis is a major problem for young people, especially girls, it reduces their self-confidence.					
3	Skeletal fluorosis severely reduces capacity for work and earning income.					

Contd...

Contd...

4	Skeletal fluorosis reduces the patient's interaction with other members of the community and leads to loneliness.					
5	Better quality drinking water would reduce skeletal fluorosis.					
6	The damage in your body due to 'fluorosis' is irreversible and no medicinal remedy for skeletal fluorosis.					
7	Is there difficulty in marriages because of dental fluorosis?					
8	Is there is inferiority complex or decrease in self-confidence?					
9	Any other problems					

Investigator's note:

Investigator's name .... Signature .... Date ......

8. DOCTOR'S QUESTIONNAIRE

Doctors Code			
D	T	V	Form No

Qs – 2. Queries from Doctors – GPs, Orthopedics, and Dentist

A. To General Practitioners

Name of the Doctor:

Address:

Telephone (LL) STD code .... No. .... (M) ....

Specialization .... No. of Years Experience ....

Since when you are practicing in this area? ....

1. How many patients you see on an average in a day. Nos. ...
2. What kind of patients you are getting? Is there any patient with following symptoms?

Joint pain	***Neck pain***	***Back pain***	***Discolored tooth***	***Others***

3. Do you think that this pain is because of fluoride in water or due to dietary factors?
4. How do you differentiate between fluorosis and MSD?
5. How many patients are you getting of fluorosis, if you can differentiate?
6. What kind of medication/treatment you provide to them?
7. Do you advise for any diagnostic tests of the followings:

Blood serum: Yes/No	***Urine: Yes/No***	***X-rays: Yes/No***	***X-ray details***	***Others***

8. Which age group patients you get more? Age in years

<6	6–12	12–18	18–40	40–60	> 60	Total (male)
<6	6–12	12–18	18–40	40–60	> 60	Total (female)

9. What kind of common signs/symptoms you are getting in patients of fluorosis?

Dental =

Skeletal =

10. Do you suggest anything about water quality, especially for fluoride?
11. Since last 3-4 years there is supply of Dharoi Dam's water in this location; do you have any knowledge no. of reporting cases [decreased or increased] of DF, MSD or of complaints of gastrointestinal [decreased or increased] cases?
12. What kind of nutrition deficiency do you find among your patients? Tell me separately for men and women and preferably with age brackets.
13. What suggestions you can give regarding mitigation of fluorosis in this area?

B. To Dentists

1. What is the average no. of patients visit your clinic in day?
2. How many patients you are getting of dental fluorosis?

	Male	***Female***	***Total***
Number			
Age in years			

3. Since last 3–4 years there is supply of Dharoi Dam's water in this location; do you have any knowledge no. of reporting cases [decreased or increased] of DF [decreased or increased] cases?
4. Do the patient seek treatment? If yes, what kind of treatment they want?

Bleaching	*Veneering*	*Crowns*	*Others*

5. How much money they would like to spend on treatment of dental fluorosis?
6. What do you advise them regarding quality of water they use?
7. What do you suggest for dental cream/paste? Tell me some of the name of tooth paste that you suggest.
8. Do you suggest any special diet to your patients? If so, what are they?
9. What suggestions you can give regarding mitigation of dental fluorosis in this area?

9. CHEMISTS/MEDICAL SHOPS QUESTIONNAIRE

Medical Shop Code			
D	T	V	Form No.

Qs – 3. Queries from Medical Shop

1. Identification of the Shop

1. Name of chemist shop ....
2. Name of respondent: ....
3. Role of respondent in shop ....
4. Opening date of shop ....
5. How long you are working in this shop? ....

2. About the Sale of Medicines

1. Do you know about Fluorosis? Yes/No ....
2. Do you sell Fluoridated toothpaste? Yes/No.......................
3. If yes, which brands? ....
4. Do you sell any Tooth Whitening product? Yes/No ...... Its quantity ....

3. Chemist/Medical Shops:

1. Which are frequently sold pain killers/Gas problems?
2. Is frequency of sale of pain killers/Gas problems changed after change in quality of water (since Dharoi water supply came)?

Sl. No.	*Name of medicines*	*Mainly used for*	*Increased*	*Decreased*	*Same*

3. Are patients coming directly for purchase of pain killers/Gas problems or through prescriptions?
4. Where do patients in your shop come from?
5. From where do most patients for pain-killers/Gas problems come from?
6. Do you keep annual records of sales of medicines? If yes, can I have access to some of the painkiller's/ Gas problems sales over past 5 years?

Investigator's Note:

Investigator's Name:......................... Signature .... Date

BIBLIOGRAPHY

BIBLIOGRAPHY

1. Mehsana Fluoride Area Health Baseline Survey; Desai, Dr (Mrs) Vikas K; Govt. Medical College, Surat. (http://www.carewater.org/fluorosisNG.pdf)
2. Fluorosis in Gujarat: A Disaster; Ahead Tushaar Shah and Rajnarayan Indu (IWMI study 2004) (http://www.carewater.org/fluorosisNG.pdf)
3. A Treatise on Fluorosis by Dr Susheela, AK; 2007
4. http://www.krassindia.org/fluoride_tre.htm © 2005 Krass India
5. Skeletal Fluorosis in India and Its Relevance to the West- Fluoride Action Network, May 2004 (http://www.fluoridealert.org/fluorosis-india.htm)
6. Fluoride in Drinking-water by J Fawell, K Bailey, J Chilton, E Dahi, L Fewtrell and Y Magara. ISBN: 1900222965. Published by IWAPublishing, London, UK, World Health Organization (WHO) 2006.
7. Reversal of Fluorosis in Children; SK Gupta, RC Gupta, AK Seth and A Gupta, Jaipur, India (Abstract from Acta Paediatrica Japonica 38 (5) 513-519 1996) (http://www.ncbi.nlm.nih.gov/pubmed/8942013)
8. The Fluoride Debate: A response to American Dental Associations Booklet, Fluoridation Facts. National survey of U.S. school children conducted by the National Institute of Dental Research, 1986-87 (http://www.fluoridedebate.com/question19.html)
9. "Understanding the Disease of Endemic Skeletal Fluorosis and Ways to Contain It" by Raja Reddy (http://www.fluorosisinandhra.org/Booklet_Fluorosis.pdf)
10. Endemic Fluorosis in Southern Rajasthan, India, By SL Choubisa Dungarpur, Rajasthan, India, Fluoride Vol. 34 No. 1 61-70 2001 Research Report 61 (http:// www.fluoride-journal.com/01-34-1/341-61.pdf)
11. Fluoride and Fluorosis (http://www.krassindia.org/downloads/ebook1.pdf)
12. http://www.fluoridealert.org/health/teeth/Fluorosis/criteria.html
13. http://en.wikipedia.org/wiki/Dental_fluorosis#Physiology
14. http://www.who.int/water_sanitation_health/diseases/fluorosis/en/
15. http://www.fluoridealert.org/s-fluorosis.htm
16. http://www.fluoridealert.org/health/teeth/fluorosis/
17. http://www.fluoridation.com/teeth.htm
18. http://www.aap.org/oralhealth/pact/ch6_sect4.cfm
19. http://www.fluorideandfluorosis.com/Diagnosis/Diagnosis.html
20. http://www.medicinaoral.com/odo/volumenes/v1i1/03.pdf
21. http://www.colgate.com/app/CP/US/EN/OC/Information/Articles/Oral-and- Dental-Health-Basics/Checkups-and-Dental- Procedures/Fluoride/article/Fluorosis.cvsp
22. http://en.wikipedia.org/wiki/Fluoride_toxicity
23. http://www.imageawareness.com/acrobat/fluoride.pdf
24. http://www.fluorideresearch.org/CFTS/files/CFTS.pdf
25. http://www.pauapress.com/fluoride/files/1418.pdf

26. http://cis.uchicago.edu/outreach/summerinstitute/2010/documents/sti2010-tata- eradication-of-fluorosis-in-india.pdf
27. http://www.earth-prints.org/bitstream/2122/2590/1/D'Alessandro_EnvTox06.pdf
28. http://www.cdc.gov/nchs/data/databriefs/db53.pdf
29. http://www.scielo.br/pdf/rpsp/v15n1/20832.pdf
30. http://www.svaindia.org/word_document/Report%20on%20fluorosis.pdf
31. http://www.medicinaoral.com/medoralfree01/v14i2/medoralv14i2p103.pdf
32. Den-1999-Biological mechanisms of dental fluorosis relevant to the use of fluoride supplements.-Community Dent Oral Epidemiol-27-41-7-http://www.healthmantra.com/REVIEWS/fluorosis.shtml
33. Rozier-1994-Epidemiologic indices for measuring the clinical manifestations of dental fluorosis: overview and critique.-Adv Dent Res-8-39-55http://www.healthmantra.com/REVIEWS/fluorosis.shtml
34. http://en.wikipedia.org/wiki/Skeletal_fluorosis
35. Fluoride and Fluorosis: about fluorosis http://www.fluorideandfluorosis.com/Fluorosis/Fluorosis.html
36. http://www.fluoridealert.org/health/bone/cellular/index.html
37. http://www.cdc.gov/fluoridation/safety/dental_fluorosis.htm
38. http://www.nofluoride.com/Unicef_fluor.cfm
39. http://healthmantra.com/ypb/apr01/fluorosis.shtml
40. http://www.ncbi.nlm.nih.gov/pmc/articles/PMC2883808/

GLOSSARY

GLOSSARY

DF = Dental Fluorosis

HHS = Households

No. = Number

MSD = Musculoskeletal Disease

VA = Gout/Arthritis in Gujarati

NA= Not Applicable/ Not Available

MDG = Millennium Development Goals

Govt. = Government

IWMI= International Water Management Institute

RO = Reverse osmosis

Vit. = Vitamin

Index

Page numbers followed by *f* refer to figure and *t* refer to table

A

Abdominal pains 18
Acute toxicity 16
Age group variation of dental fluorosis 60
Ascorbic acid 35
Awareness of drinking water 66, 87

B

Bloated feeling 18
Blood in stool 18
Brittle nails 18

C

Chemobiokinetics and metabolism of fluoride 11
Chronic
  fatigue 17
  toxicity 17
Classification of dental fluorosis 56*t*
Common dental diseases 10
Community education and mobilization 34
Comparative analysis with IWMI study 69
Composite bonding 34
Constipation 18, 65
Creating disease awareness 33
Crippling fluorosis 31

D

Dean's index criteria for dental fluorosis 79
Dental
  caries 10, 28, 29*f*
  fluorosis 10, 19, 19*f*, 20, 21, 25*f*, 27-29, 29*f*, 43, 50, 56, 58, 69, 75, 76
Determine dental fluorosis 23*f*
Diarrhea 18, 65
Discoloration of teeth with pattern 23
Domestic defluoridation 36
Dryness of throat and excessive water consumption 17

E

Effect of fluoride
  concentration on teeth 14*t*
  toxicity on human health 15*t*
Enamel fluorosis 20
Endemic fluorosis 44
Excessive nervousness 18
Excretion of fluorides 13

F

Feeling of nausea 18
Fluoride 3
  and bone cells 14*f*
  and diabetes 32
  and thyroid 32
  concentration 14
  in toothpaste 16
  in water 4
  toxicity 15
Fluorosis 1, 5, 6, 19, 42
  diagnostic tests 32, 33
  photographs 75

G

Gastrointestinal
  disturbances 17
  problems 32
Geochemistry of fluorine 1
Grades of
  dental fluorosis 25, 60
    in different age groups 62*t*
  fluorosis 24

H

Headaches 17
Health education 33
Hydrogen fluoride 11
Hydroxyapatite 3

K

KRASS defluoridation process 38

M

Male infertility 18
Mental work capacity 32
Mild
  dental fluorosis 25*f*
  fluorosis 56
Moderate
  dental fluorosis 25
  fluorosis 56
Muscles spasms 17
Muscular
  manifestations 32
  weakness 17
Musculoskeletal
  disorders 62
  fluorosis 62, 75, 76, 85

N

Nalgonda process 37
Non-communicable disease 42
Non-skeletal manifestations 32

P

Periodontal disease 10
Porcelain laminate veneers 35*f*
Prevalence of
  dental fluorosis 58*t*
    in different age groups 60*t*
Preventing dental fluorosis 35
Pyorrhea 10

Q

Quantification of fluoride toxicity on human health 15

R

Renal insufficiency 20
Repeated miscarriages or still births 18
Reversal of fluorosis in children 42

S

Severe
  dental fluorosis 24, 24*f*, 25
  fluorosis 56
Severity of dental fluorosis 34
Six types of fluorosis 28
Skeletal fluorosis 30, 31
Symptoms of chronic fluoride poisoning 17

T

Tenderness in stomach area 18
Thyroid stimulating hormone 33
Tooth whitening 34
Treatment of
  acute toxicity 17
  fluorosis 34
Turner's hypoplasia 10
Types of fluorosis 28*f*

U

Urinary tract irritation 17

V

Vitamin C 35, 81

W

Water
  harvesting 39
  supply 53, 83